# WEIGHT LOSS *for* AFRICAN-AMERICAN WOMEN

# WEIGHT LOSS
## *for* AFRICAN-AMERICAN WOMEN

## AN EIGHT-WEEK GUIDE *to* BETTER HEALTH

*George Edmond Smith, M.D., M.Ed.*

HILTON PUBLISHING COMPANY • ROSCOE, ILLINOIS

ISBN 0–9675258–5–3

Copyright © 2001 by George Edmond Smith

Hilton Publishing Company
PO Box 737, Roscoe, IL 61073
815-885-1070
www.hiltonpub.com

Cover photos: left © Ariel Skelley/Corbis Stock Market; center © Jose Luis Pelaez Inc./Corbis Stock Market; right © George Shelley/Corbis Stock Market.

### Publisher's Cataloging-in-Publication
*(Provided by Quality Books, Inc.)*

Smith, George Edmond.
    Eight Weeks to better health : weight los for African American women / Edmond Smith — 1st ed.
    p. cm.
    Includes bibliographical references and index.
    ISBN: 0–9675258–5–3

    1. Weight loss. 2. African American women—Health and hygiene. I. Title.

RM222.2.S65 2001                  613.7'045
                                      QBI01–201011

Printed and bound in the United States of America

## DEDICATION AND ACKNOWLEDGMENTS

Brenda Ford, my life-partner, helped make this book sensitive to the needs of Black women and indeed of every woman who has ever challenged herself to a better quality of life. Without her help and her unconditional love, I could never have written this book.

I would also like to thank Elizabeth Curtis for the insight, talent, and most of all, sensitivity she lent to the book

Finally, my warm gratitude to Eileen Folk for her wonderful, healthy recipes and to M. Jackson for his eye-catching illustrations.

# Contents

## PART ONE • BACKGROUND

*Introduction* 3

*Chapter 1 • How We Got This Way* 11

*Chapter 2 • Reclaiming Your Self* 19

*Chapter 3 • Why Is Family Medicine So Important to Women's Health and Weight Loss?* 29

*Chapter 4 • Emotional Fitness* 37

*Chapter 5 • Health Literacy and Motivation* 49

## PART TWO • SISTERHOOD CONNECTIONS: THE JOURNEY

*Chapter 6 • Four Women* 63

*Chapter 7 • Week One* 79

*Chapter 8 • Week Two* 93

*Chapter 9 • Week Three* 105

*Chapter 10 • Week Four* 115

*Chapter 11 • Week Five* 125

*Chapter 12 • Week Six* 139

*Chapter 13 • Week Seven* 155

*Chapter 14 • Week Eight* 163

## PART THREE • TOOLS FOR THE JOURNEY

*Chapter 15 • Diagnosing Your Own Eating Disorders* 173

Emotional Fitness Inventory • Physical Inventory
Social Inventory • Stress Inventory

*Chapter 16 • Meditation* 183

*Chapter 17 • Healthy Ways to Think and Act* 191

*Chapter 18 • Eight-Week Sample Meal Plan* 199

Sample Meal Plans • Sample Weekly Menus
Starch and Bread List • Fruit List • Vegetable List • Milk List
Meat List • Fat Exchange List • Free Food List

*Chapter 19 • Calculating Your Daily Calories and BMI
(Body Mass Index)* 249

*Appendix A • Additional Exercises* 251

*Appendix B • Planners, Logs, and Lists* 257

Meal Planner • Daily Food Diary • Aerobic Activity Log
Strength Training Log • Healthy Grocery List

*Appendix C • Recipes for Healthy Living* 265

*Appendix D • Resources for Good Health* 329

*References* 353

*Subject Index* 358

*Recipe Index* 366

*Part One*

# BACKGROUND

# Introduction

*In search of my mother's garden, I found my own.*
*—Alice Walker*

THIS ISN'T JUST ANOTHER DIET BOOK. Diets come and go, but in this book I'm interested in what blossoms forever. This book means to strengthen you own experience of a self that knows the power of love. You'll find that that experience is the beginning of riches.

If dieting could make you happy, you'd think that all fashion models would be ecstatic. But actually, many of them are plagued with eating disorders, just like far too many of the rest of us. What gives happiness is coming into touch with your full self, body and soul. It's toward that happiness that this book offers to take you.

The key words and phrases you will read in this book are:

- Wellness
- Life choices
- Personal journey
- Integration
- Wholeness
- Personhood
- Empowerment

A fulfilling life depends on your understanding of wellness and the actions you take toward achieving it. Wellness is the motivating force for becoming a healthier you. As you place wellness within your personal sanctuary, you will begin to create an image of your mind, body, and spirit merging, making you feel whole, and yes, well.

Feminist Alice Walker coined the term *womanist* to describe women of color who are committed to the survival and wholeness of all people, both male and female. What a powerful word it is. The strength underlying this word is what Black women everywhere innately possess. Being committed to yourself requires only the strength that is already an exceptional part of you. A colleague of Walker's, Delores Williams, could not have been more clear when she said that "it is so important that you love yourself, regardless." This book is about just that.

Even four hundred years before the birth of Jesus, the ancient philosophers were speaking of wellness. Hippocrates once said:

> All parts of the body that have a function, if used in modera-
> tion, and exercised in labors to which each is accustomed,
> become healthy and well developed and age slowly; but if
> unused and left idle, they become liable to disease, defective in
> growth and age quickly.

One might think that the philosopher's important message would have woven its way into the fabric of our lifestyles over such a long time, but the truth is that for most Americans it has not. A lack of time in a hurried world, coupled with our need for convenience, has interfered with this ideal. But now I want to revive it for you, my beautiful Black sisters.

It is no secret that African American women are far more likely than other groups of women to die of serious diseases. Many of these diseases are either attributed to or made worse by carrying too much weight on a body frame designed to hold less. Fatalities caused by heart disease are 70 percent higher for Black women than for any other group of women, and more Black women than ever are developing disabling diabetes, especially Type II. For both diseases, being a great deal overweight is the most serious risk factor. Consider these troubling facts:

- One in ten Black women over the age of forty is more than 100 pounds overweight.
- Black women who are severely overweight are more prone to die of endometrial, cervical, and breast cancer than women who are not seriously overweight.
- Black women are also at risk for pulmonary disease, gout, and arthritis if they are seriously overweight.

In Philadelphia, for example, nearly 60 percent of the six thousand deaths in 1994 were Black women who died from heart disease and complications arising from diabetes. More alarming is that *Black women made up less than 25 percent of the city's population.* This doesn't mean you can't celebrate your roundness, but it does mean that being too round may cause you to die too soon.

The Center for Disease Control (CDC) in Atlanta, Georgia, has now proclaimed obesity to be "an epidemic of enormous proportion and impact." And the Presidential Health Commission has pronounced obesity as the number-one health problem facing all Americans. Reclaiming your health and taking ownership of your personal journey is the only way to reverse the consequences of a sedentary, convenience-filled lifestyle. In order to combat this alarming, detrimental health trend, *Weight Loss for African American Women: Eight Weeks to Better Health* offers proven tools that will help you make positive life choices and change unhealthy behavior patterns before it's too late.

As an African American family doctor, I see women of color struggle with the unhealthy effects of carrying too much weight, which is why I have written this book. Because empowerment of Black women in all areas of life is my ultimate goal, I have included not only the physical aspects of caring for the self but the mental, emotional, spiritual, intellectual, and social wellness components as well. You may have already seen doctors who provide only a strict, medical approach to healthcare and who don't see you as a whole person with feelings, thoughts, and emotions. This is why the "You need to lose weight" statements don't ever work.

Countless hours of television, magazine, and billboard advertising promising quick and easy weight loss are causing many of you to see yourselves as unacceptable. In fact, 75 percent of American women are dissatisfied with their appearance. That, in itself, is a travesty. Because of the constant pressure to live up to some unattainable societal ideal, too many of you are caught up in the myth that if you eat fewer calories, you will lose weight. The result is that the human body goes into starvation mode, holding on to every ounce of energy from the little bit of food you do eat. This is why the calorie-limiting diets recommended by many physicians simply do not work. By relying on a purely medical model, they ignore the equally important emotional, spiritual, and social aspects of a woman's life.

As you will soon learn in your journey toward wellness, you can eat, eat, eat, as long as you do it intelligently. The aim is not to stop eating but to be fit and energetic, and to enjoy better health. To those of you who have grown accustomed to today's sedentary lifestyle, that's the better option this book offers. To those who are already taking care of yourselves, this book will introduce additional ways for you to focus on your well-being.

Change is never easy, especially when you've been doing things the same way all of your life. But becoming healthier, rather than focusing specifically on weight loss, is a very powerful incentive for the women whom you will read about in this book. Their stories will empower and encourage you.

It is no secret that in the United States alone, people spend more than $30 billion annually on weight loss programs, gimmicks, and fads. Yet, I believe you are tired of placing your trust in diet books that profess quick fixes and are void of any cultural sensitivity to the Black woman's pride in her roundness. Slim is not "in" within the Black community, but I'm sure you will agree that being healthy should be. As strong African American women, you are dedicated to the robustness of our culture and deserve a wellness plan that will work for you, one that is honest, inviting, and practical for your lifestyle.

In these pages, you will not find quick fixes or torturous methods of becoming fit. There are no recipes for magic diet cookies although there are a couple of good ones for chocolate chip and oatmeal raisin. Giving up food is as unappealing as a long day of working overtime.

Although I present a medical model of obesity and an integrated weight loss program, I also emphasize how your mental, emotional, spiritual, intellectual, and social well-being can help you achieve wellness. One specific example of this occurred when one of my favorite patients made a bet with me after I suggested that losing weight would relieve her lower back pain. She smiled, and emphatically told me that she was not overweight and that her husband liked her that way, even though her 5' 6" frame held well over 280 pounds. I showed her how physicians determine what "too much weight" is by using the Body Mass Index (BMI), discussed in later chapters. It revealed severe obesity, which was a serious threat to her overall wellness and quality of life. The only way her back would stop hurting, I told her, was if she lost the excess weight. Needless to say, even though I won the initial bet, she was the ultimate winner. Her name is Diane, and she agreed to become a part of this book. You will meet her in a later chapter.

Balance is a necessary part of wellness, and it takes effort to make it an essential part of your life. As strong Black women, you have the power within yourselves to contribute to your own personal healing. This book follows four women who learned to become more balanced through community building and integration of their personalities, shedding unwanted pounds in the process. Their personal journeys are the most poignant part of this book because they are true. The women in the stories vary in age, amount of weight lost, lifestyle, income, and educational level. They share a common thread, however: the motivation to achieve their goal through helping each other. You will identify with them. Now is the time to give yourself permission to explore all of your avenues of expression, and become a healthier version of yourself.

Yes, you should "love yourself, regardless," but something has to change in order for you to become the healthy version of yourself. Black women who are severely overweight are health limited, and their quality of life suffers as a result. Certainly, losing weight and keeping it off is a challenge, but this book will challenge you with still deeper invitations to change, and show you that change is within your power.

What makes this book different from others is that not only does it include an in-depth understanding of African American culture and eating habits, it also deals specifically with ways to recognize personality traits that may keep you from attaining your goal, whether it's losing weight to become healthier or some other goal.

Becoming goal oriented is always the first step in anyone's journey toward better health. Most Black women already possess this naturally; it simply needs to be activated. Stress most impedes the process of setting goals. Working long hours with no time to concentrate on your own needs, making sure your children's needs are met, or meeting the needs of family members can put a damper on thinking about yourself. Americans in general, and American women in particular, find themselves too busy in this sped-up world, but the problem appears to be even worse for Black women. You do a great deal for others while sacrificing your own well-being; it's time to acknowledge that you should now come first. Only by keeping yourselves physically and emotionally strong can you be of real help to others.

As a physician, I have heard many reasons why Black women are not anxious to become healthier. The most common are "I have no time" or "I need to lose weight before I go to a gym; I'm ashamed to be seen in shorts with this body" or "I simply have no energy to exercise." Many of these statements can be attributed to feeling imbalanced in different areas of your life.

Imagine for a moment a pie with five slices to it, slices that correspond to the major parts of our personality. Let's say the five slices of the pie represent the following areas of your life:

- Emotional/mental
- Physical/sexual
- Intellectual
- Social
- Spiritual

It is important for each slice to be as equal in proportion as possible because each area works in conjunction with the others to balance your personality. It is this balance that makes you happy and that gives you the energy and motivation to accomplish your goals. If one slice is missing, unhappiness and emotional fatigue can occur.

Balance ensures happiness and contentment, providing the energy you need to stay motivated. Because I am a physician dedicated to Black women's health, I know that you live in a world that often seems unfair and filled with overwhelming stress. This book is designed to help you achieve and keep your balance despite such pressures. Using a personal inventory checklist, this book takes you on a tour of your personality and emotional fitness, and teaches you how to assess unhealthy patterns that keep you stuck.

The book provides other tools for living as well, including:

- Self-tests on personality, emotional fitness, and stress. What parts of your personality are unbalanced? And how does your emotional fitness affect your ability to stay healthy and happy? Are you able to effectively manage stress?
- A personalized weight loss program and overall assessment of what your personal needs are based on your personality and emotional fitness. This guide will help you to work out a program of better physical, mental, emotional, spiritual, and intellectual health. Lifestyle changes are custom designed to meet your individual needs.
- Approaches to motivation that keep you goal oriented instead of trapped, and show you how to break the cycle of yo-yo dieting and prevent it from starting up again once it's under control.
- Sensitivity to cultural issues that affect African American women and ways to cultivate a "me first" attitude using the various aspects of your personality.
- Real stories from African American women who have lost weight using a community-building approach and why losing weight was important to them; obstacles that they faced daily, as well as a primer on the basic nutrients and how to manipulate them to fit your lifestyle.
- Handsome drawings of exercises, food charts, personal logs, and graphics that demonstrate how the "personality pie" works.

I recommend that you browse through the resources in Part Three while you are reading Parts One and Two. The resources show you in detail how to move forward in your own journey. (Chapter 18, for instance, will show you how to plan menus for the opening weeks of your diet. You'll discover that healthy food doesn't have to be tasteless.)

Finding your own "personal garden" can be one of the most rewarding experiences in your life, and it's time to do just that. Keep in mind that although food is at the center of this book, you are not defined by the foods you eat. You have been living a certain way for a long time. Finding your own garden of success does not just mean you should change the way you eat; it goes beyond this. It is something deep and personal inside you; it is the way you think and feel.

Eating habits in the African American home have prevailed for years, if not for generations, through family tradition. Black-eyed peas and greens saturated with pork fat have been served at family gatherings for a long time, haven't they? How do you, as an African American woman who has eaten like this for years, change your habits? I answer that question helpfully and honestly, understanding that it's not easy to change a lifetime of bad habits like eating high-fat foods or smoking, not even when someone tells you that if you don't change you will die. Eating, after all, has become part of the deeper fabric of our lives. We celebrate around food, we meet around food, we wed around food, and we mourn around food.

Still, you can change. If I didn't believe that—indeed, if I didn't believe in *you*—I wouldn't have written this book. As a passionate African American woman, you are savvy about your life. You know what you want, when you want it, and how you want it. So read on, the women in this book are just like you. The only difference is that they learned to make themselves the center of their world. You deserve the same!

# Chapter 1

## How We Got This Way

*Never forget the importance of history. To know nothing of what happened before you took your place on earth is to remain a child for ever and ever.*
*—Author unknown*

WOMEN OF AFRICAN DESCENT have created and maintained families; communities; sisterhoods; unions; and religious, social, and political organizations. All have been instrumental in fostering both the individual and collective good, and nurturing the continuing development of African American cultural forms. This is especially true regarding the culture of food. Most of our beliefs about food are conditioned by our African origins, upheld through hundreds of years of tradition.

Did you know that every time you spread peanut butter on your bread, you are eating African food? Peanuts and peanut paste are staple foods of Africa and were brought to the United States by slaves. The origins of boiled peanuts, okra, and black-eyed peas are also African. Did you also know that an African American named George Washington Carver invented peanut butter?

"Soul food" descended from slave cooking, from famine and want. Slave cooking used greens, beans, and the parts of the pig rejected at the plantation house, such as pig's knuckles, tripe, hog maws, and ears. Since many slaves were given only corn rations to survive on, these parts were used to supplement the slave's meager pantry. Wild game such as squirrel and possum also figured among the meats used. Catfish, trout, and shrimp were dominant among the fish. Since tools for cooking were sparse and time was limited, only one pot was used to prepare soul food.

Every ethnic group has what it calls soul food—soothing comfort food that brings back warm memories of family dinners. Today, in America, the term *soul food* simply means African American cuisine. To fully understand the concept of soul food, you must learn the traditional foods of Africa. Many common American foods are indigenous to Africa. Grains, legumes, yams, sorghum, watermelon, pumpkin, okra, and leafy greens could be found as early as 4000 B.C. on the African continent. Eggplant, cucumber, onion, and garlic are believed to be of African origin, and a small number of fruits are grown on the continent: wild lemons, oranges, dates, and figs.

Culinary historians believe that at the beginning of the fourteenth century, around the time of early European exploration, explorers brought their own food supplies and introduced them into the African diet. Such foods as turnips, from Morocco, and cabbage, from Spain, would later play an important part in the history of African American cuisine.

The average African ate a mostly vegetarian diet; meat was used lightly to flavor greens. Seafood showed up often in stews, usually served with a starch. Okra and native peppers were used as seasoning, and salt as a preservative. Research scientist William Bascom discovered that a large number of tribal Africans shared basic cooking techniques. Simplicity was the trademark. Utensils for cooking and eating were made from earthenware or prepared gourds or other squashes. Africans often fried foods in palm oil or vegetable butters, toasted and roasted using fire, and baked in ashes. Some ingredients were smoked for flavoring, and others thickened with nuts and seeds. Africans also made rice dishes and created fritters.

A common African meal consisted of rice, chicken, and milk while the poorest Africans ate a type of couscous with leafy vegetables. This made the African diet healthy and satisfying. The tradition of communal living and shared meals was the perfect environment for conversation, reciting oral history, and storytelling.

When slave trading began in the early 1400s, the diet of newly enslaved Africans changed on the long journeys from their homeland. On these terrible voyages across the Atlantic Ocean, small portions of rice and beans, with the occasional vegetable or piece of fruit, replaced their normally healthy diet. A "slabber" sauce, made from old beef and rotten fish and salt, was poured over the rice and beans in an attempt to fill the slaves' stomachs.

Some of the indigenous crops of Africa later began showing up in the slaves' new home in the Americas. Tales of seeds from watermelons, okras, and sesame being transported in a slave's ears, hair, or clothing could be true. The more likely explanation is that the European slave traders, urged by the Africans themselves, brought the food over for trade. Whatever the case, these familiar foods would soon become part of America's southern crops.

Remarkably, some African slaves actually had a better diet than their owners did. The owners ate mostly fatty foods, with little or no vegetables and lots of sweets and alcohol that left them lethargic. The slaves needed to be strong and energetic to work the fields, so large vegetarian meals were encouraged and drinking discouraged. Iced tea and lemonade became typical drinks. As the Africans began to assimilate into the American slave society, they made do with the ingredients at hand. The fresh vegetables found in Africa were replaced by the throwaway foods from the plantation house. Their vegetables were the tops of turnips and beets and dandelions. Soon the African slaves were cooking with new types of greens: collards, kale, cress, mustard, and pokeweed. With a lot of lard for flavor from a slaughtered hog and cracklings from its skin, it made for a filling meal. Plantation owners gave out weekly rations of corn meal, and a few pounds of meat and black molasses from the smokehouse. The women would use these ingredients, with onions, garlic, thyme, and bay leaf, to create a variety of dishes. Cornmeal was turned into bread. Meat (pig's feet, ham hocks, chitterlings, pig ears, hog jowl, tripe, and cracklings), along with generous portions of greens, became the main dish. The molasses and cornmeal were mixed to become a dessert.

The slave diet began to evolve when slaves entered the plantation houses as cooks. With an array of new ingredients at their fingertips and a well-tuned African palate, the cooks made delectable foods for the plantation owners. Suddenly, southern cooking took on new meaning. Fried chicken began to appear on the tables, sweet potatoes (which had replaced the African yam) sat next to the boiled white potato. Regional foods like apples, peaches, berries, nuts, and grains soon became puddings and pies. Possum was the meat of choice among slaves because hunting was done during the only free hours a slave had after all the work for their master was complete, in the wee hours of the night. Soon the slave's cuisine became known as "good times" food.

Because each state had its own cultural influences, the African dishes began to take on the qualities of those states. Rich, saucy dishes with a French accent came from Louisiana; Carolina's Spanish culture introduced dishes like jambalaya and a strange food called sausage. A bouillabaisse or a cassoulet, found in French cuisine, were changed by slaves into a gumbo using shellfish from the bayou, okra, and fish filets to make a dish more to the liking of African taste buds. Unlike dishes from other countries, with names that usually suggested the ingredients, Black cuisine had names that did not necessarily hint at the ingredients, but did offer a little history of how it came about:

- The hushpuppy got its name from the dredgings and catfish scraps that otherwise would have been thrown out. Being thrifty, the cook would send the fish down to the slave quarters where the women added a little milk, egg, and onion, and fried it up. It is said these cakes were sometimes tossed at the dogs to keep them quiet while the food was being transferred from the pot to the table, hence, "Hush puppy!"
- Hoecakes are a dish said to have been a corn bread batter that was heaped onto a spade or hoe, and held over the open fire to make a quick bread.
- Ashcakes are a corn meal mixture baked in an open fire. The baked bread is then washed after cooking and served.
- A "gut strut" is another name for a big pot of chittlins.

No matter the stories, Black cuisine was wholesome and frugal; every ingredient available was used. Nothing was ever wasted in the

Black kitchen. Leftover fish became croquettes (by adding an egg, cornmeal or flour, and seasonings, then breaded and deep-fried). Stale bread became bread pudding. Even the liquid from the boiled vegetables was turned into "pot likker" and used as a type of gravy or as a drink in itself. While the master would have an apple, peach, or cherry pie, slaves produced fried pies that could be tucked into a pocket for a sweet pick-me-up in the fields.

The heartiness of oil filled the slave's stomachs and provided energy for a long day on the plantation. Black women traditionally prepared the food, and they never followed a recipe. Ingenuity turned scraps into delicious, hearty, satisfying meals.

There are no records that show exactly how many of our African ancestors died during or after their journey to the New World, or what brutality they endured on the slave ships and beyond, but the stress they suffered most certainly caused physiological changes in their bodies, something that can still be seen in our population today. We carry the genes of our ancestors, and foods that were high in saturated fat and salt were, and still are, staples in our daily eating patterns. During times of starvation or limited food intake, our bodies learned to metabolize those foods that were rich in calories. The reason? We expended more energy, and our bodies were able to keep shedding excess calories. This is also a major reason that obesity and associated diseases like diabetes were not common.

Our ancestors adjusted to other ordeals as well. They survived hard toil in heat and humidity because their kidneys became conditioned to hold onto salt (sodium) and consequently water. Further, their bodies were under stress, and therefore subject to excess cortisol secretions into their bloodstreams. Cortisol causes water retention. We are our ancestor's progeny; their minds and bodies are ours.

Eating foods high in calories and low in nutrition continued for generations. Following the Emancipation Proclamation and into the period of the Industrial Revolution and the Gilded Age, family members became more scattered, and so as not to lose contact with others, Sunday dinners became a time for families to get together. It was common for a son or daughter to travel some distance just for a good home-cooked meal. Aunts, uncles, cousins (both real and pretend) would converge for a meal, not on the largest home, but on the house with the best cook.

Even though our ancestors became free, they still maintained the patterns of eating unhealthy foods. Unwanted portions of meats found their way to the plates of African American families. They were cheap, easy to find, and became a part of the African American culture. Eating fatty meats and cooking with lard would be euphemized as soul food in the twentieth century and passed down through generations, persisting today.

The Great Depression contributed much to determining what kinds of foods African Americans used as a foundation for their diets. Not only did women who prepared meals during that time look for the least expensive meats, they started to prepare potatoes, pasta, rice, and large amounts of bread to fill their families' stomachs. The trend toward eating sizeable portions of starchy carbohydrates and few fresh vegetables began. During this period, women were forced to work like their husbands to forge a living.

Although industrial labor was intense and repetitive, it did not provide the same physical benefits that working on a farm did. African Americans also did not have the same leisure time that white America had, which produced additional stress. African Americans became heavier, and diseases that affected the heart and that caused diabetes began to surface.

In the mid-1960s, when the civil rights movement was just beginning, terms like "soul man," "soulful," and "soul," were used in connection with African Americans. It caught on in mainstream America, and someone coined the term *soul food* for Black cuisine. Today, when most people think of soul food, they see a table heavy with trays of watermelon, ribs, candied sweet potatoes or yams, greens, and fried chicken. Still, we can see some signs of change. Black-owned restaurants have begun to offer healthier versions of traditional foods, and excellent lowfat soul food cookbooks are on the market. (See, for example, the selections from *The New Soul Food Cookbook* by Wilbert Jones, reprinted in *The Heart of the Matter: The African American's Guide to Heart Disease, Heart Treatment, and Heart Wellness* by Hilton M. Hudson, M.D. and Herbert Stern, Ph.D. [Hilton Publishing].)

The upshot is that over the past fifty years, technological advancements have changed things for the better, but our lives are different, less physical. We are just too busy to spend hours in the kitchen cooking up the traditional foods of our ancestors, and if we do have the time, we are not taking the steps necessary to rework those old recipes into healthier versions to benefit ourselves. The dilemma facing us is that we still tend to eat as we did hundreds of years ago, yet now we consume more calories in our daily diets than we expend in our daily activities.

Recent research reveals another problem as well—one especially important to Black women. According to a study by researchers at the University of Pennsylvania Medical Center, overweight women of color, when they are at rest, burn fewer calories than overweight white women. The findings, published in *Obesity Research* (Vol. 5, No. 1, January 1997), are among the first to suggest that biological factors may be partly responsible for higher rates of obesity in Black women. Such a finding would provide an even more important reason for African American women to live healthier lifestyles.

Statistics show that though nearly 50 percent of Black women are overweight, they tend to lose less weight in structured weight control programs. "Although environmental factors such as diet, physical activity, and cultural preferences of body shapes are important, biological factors should be considered when trying to understand weight and weight loss in Black women," says lead author Gary D. Foster, Ph.D., clinical director of Penn's Weight and Eating Disorders Program.

Maybe when we know more about genes and how they work, we will know more about why we are the way we are. Solution-oriented Black women can accept the historical accounts about how weight became a problem, and can help change what happens to future generations of Black women.

You can speed up your metabolism and change the eating patterns that you've become accustomed to by understanding your history and then moving toward a new and different future. This book tells you how to do just that. Read on and allow me to illustrate how four women did it, using the idea of community as their driving force. They reinvented themselves, and you can, too.

# Two

## RECLAIMING YOUR SELF

*It is the mind that makes the body.*
*—Soujourner Truth*

THIS CHAPTER IS DEDICATED to two women who took care of everyone else in their lives, but not themselves—my mother, Ethel Smith, and Ms. Winnie Brown.

I met Winnie Brown a few years ago in my southwest Philadelphia medical office. For years, she had trouble following the treatment plans of other doctors. When I met her, I thought I would be able to help her since my approach to women of color is both culturally sensitive and pragmatic. Ms. Brown was a forty-year-old woman who suffered from diabetes, high blood pressure, and severe obesity. She weighed over 280 pounds. Her weight compounded her poor medical condition and made it difficult for her to even walk, but she was delightful, with an open, rather humorous personality. Ms. Brown didn't seem to mind the fact that other doctors told her she was a difficult patient. When I saw her, one hot Wednesday afternoon, she hadn't taken her medicine in two days. Although a normal blood pressure is about 120 over 70, Ms. Brown's was 210 over 130. Her blood sugar level was over 300, when it should have been no more than 100.

"Ms. Brown," I said concerned, "why didn't you take your medicine?"

Her quick response was, "Well, doctor, it's like this. I have a daughter who is twenty years old. She has a little baby boy and is having problems with her boyfriend, so she's staying with me. All the money I have goes to them, and I just don't have money to buy my medicine."

I really couldn't hold my unrest at her answer and said, "Doesn't she work? How come you didn't come here and get some samples that we keep for this type of situation?"

She didn't look at me when she said, "I didn't have time, doctor, and thought I could wait. And no, she doesn't have a job, so I have to help her. Her sister don't want nothin' to do with her because she uses that crack."

"Ms. Brown, you have to start thinking of yourself first here. You aren't going to be any help to anyone if you don't take care of yourself. Your condition is threatening your life. People here love you, and they want the best for you. You simply can't go on like this."

She started crying and promised she would change. I felt her emotion and was saddened that I had made her cry. She must have read my mind because she said, "Doctor, don't worry, it's not your fault. I know I need to be more responsible. It's just that it's all I can do to get by."

Even though Ms. Brown was sorry, she was also prone to twisting things so they kept her from making changes. She had a history of crying for the doctors she visited and telling them she would do things differently, almost always convincing her other healthcare workers that she would shortly change her tune and follow her treatment goals. I honestly thought she was doing it again, but was willing to give her the benefit of doubt. I walked her to our pharmacy to get the medication, gave her some insulin, and had her promise me that she would see me the following Monday. I thought about Ms. Brown all weekend and even told my wife about how she was like my mother, caring about everyone else but not herself.

On Monday, I arrived at my office early and noticed a large man dressed in black clothes was waiting to see me. My secretary informed me that the man wanted me to sign something. He was the funeral director of the local funeral home. Ms. Brown had died that Sunday night of a heart attack, and he wanted me to sign the death certificate. It was one of the rare times that I cried. Three months later, my staff informed me that Ms. Brown's daughter, who had taken advantage of her, had turned the house into a "crack house."

Then there is the story of my own mother. She was morbidly obese and fell victim to a minor illness that she neglected and that had escalated into severe internal infection. Owing to a complication from diabetes, she had a debilitating stroke and passed away at eighty-two years of age, after many years of being unable to communicate with the rest of the world. My mother didn't take care of herself; she always put off exercise and medical care, and ignored eating a proper diet. My mother's illness and subsequent death shaped the course of my life. It was then that I decided to devote myself to bringing quality care and education to the African American community, particularly to Black women.

My need to help Black women is clearly a result of my mother's ill health. She, like Ms. Brown and many of you who are reading this book, sacrificed her own needs while devoting much of her life to meeting her family's needs. It was my mother who took care of us, making sure that we went to the doctor even though she did not go often enough herself.

Even though she took us to our activities and encouraged us to participate in organized sports, she did not exercise. Nor was good nutrition a priority for her. Rather, she stretched every dollar as far as it would go, and that meant we didn't always eat the healthiest foods.

My mother lived for several years with an amputated leg and dementia from multiple strokes. I'm not even sure she was able to understand me when I said, "I'm sorry, I wish I could have done something to help you." She will never hear me again, but it's my hope that other Black women will.

## KNOWING YOURSELF

"Know thyself," advised an inscription on the ancient Temple of Apollo at Delphi. But what is it you know when you know yourself? How do you gain this knowledge, and what should you do with it? These questions are at the core of your personality.

Some people may answer them by seeing life as a play in which we put on different faces or play different roles for various audiences. In fact, the word *personality* comes from the Latin root *persona,* meaning "mask." The impression we make on others—or the mask we present to the world—determines how people feel about us, and in turn, how we tend to feel about ourselves from the feedback we receive from our social world.

Our everyday "performances" have a profound effect on our lives, so it pays to understand how others see us. But are the acts we put on for others an indication of who we really are? Do our outward behaviors reflect our true personalities? A complete picture of our personalities requires us to look at *all* the different parts of ourselves and to understand how each part contributes to who we are.

Reclaiming the self simply means knowing who you are, embracing every part that is you, and most important, loving and taking care of yourself. It is also the art of both empowering yourself and helping others do the same. In the process of reclaiming your self, you learn to train the voice that is uniquely yours, as well as your body, intuition, and mind.

Women should reclaim themselves because, by doing so, they learn to deepen their strength (as individuals and as a community), to voice their concerns about the world in which they live, and to bring to bear a vision for women of color. It is through a collective effort that mountains can be moved and battles can be won.

Sometimes patients tell me that their lives expand and diminish from day to day. They tell me they think talking about their weight, even to me, their physician, somehow changes them in my eyes. What most women who come to see me don't realize is that I don't measure them in terms of weight gain or loss. I approach them in terms of how well they take care of themselves and how strongly they control their lives.

Before you can become healthier yourself, it is important that you move beyond judgments of others and come to a greater acceptance of who you are. The time has come for you to reclaim the essence of who you truly are—to take a step back from the fast pace of your daily life and connect more deeply with self and spirit, and with other people.

When you connect with your deeper nature, when you know the

truth of your nature and are able to express it, you move closer to your authentic self and live a life of soul—where life, not your weight, expresses who you are. Living more authentically and creatively stimulates not only better health but also more intimate relationships and, ultimately, overall joy.

Putting yourself first is difficult, isn't it? It's okay to say yes because it's true for anyone who cares about others. Women, especially women of color, have been socialized to be the cornerstone of the family, sacrificing their own needs to care for loved ones. It is easy to understand how hard it can be to begin focusing on yourself. Cultivating a "me first" attitude without taking away from your daily, personal obligations can produce anxiety and be downright difficult. But there's a truth to hold you steady through the difficulties: *if you don't take care of yourself, you will not be able to take care of anyone else.*

Don't fool yourself into thinking you'll start taking care of yourself next week, or on New Years Day, like so many others. The time is here and now. Don't be afraid of who you are and what you are capable of. Fear itself can become a self-fulfilling prophecy; it can limit your potential. Step out on faith and take it one day at a time. Remember, losing weight is only part of the process. Little steps add up to big ones. Good decisions add up to better ones.

## KEEPING A JOURNAL AND OBSERVING YOUR THOUGHTS

Reclaiming yourself involves an awareness of thoughts, rational thinking, and constant self-affirmation. Thought awareness is the first step in the process because you cannot counter negative emotions unless you acknowledge that they exist.

Prior to beginning any physical health program, you should observe your thoughts for a time, especially when you're under stress. Avoiding unpleasant or stressful thoughts may be your normal reaction to stressful situations. This is called "stuffing." In the end, it leads to negative self-talk and sometimes even to a sense of chaos and despair.

This is why keeping a journal is essential. It helps you pay attention to negative thoughts, for only by noticing them can you change them. Because these thoughts normally appear and disappear throughout the course of the day, they are barely noticeable. Common negative thoughts might include:

- Worries about how you appear to other people
- Preoccupation with the symptoms of stress
- Dwelling on consequences of poor performance
- Self-criticism
- Feelings of inadequacy
- Feelings of not getting anywhere

Make note of such thoughts on your journey to wellness. When you are able to step away and view them objectively, you may find that little by little they come to seem less terrible and more manageable.

When you become aware of a negative thought, write it down and review it. Often, when you challenge your original notion of reality, you will see it as solvable. You will probably find it helpful to counter negative thoughts with positive affirmations. Positive self-talk builds confidence and can even motivate you. Remember, when you feel positive about the person you are, you will be inclined to place your own needs first.

Examples of positive affirmations are:

- I can do this.
- I can achieve my goals.
- I am completely myself, and people will like me for myself.
- I am completely in control of my life.
- I learn from my mistakes. They increase the basis of experience.
- I am a good and valued person in my own right.

Bringing your negative thoughts into the light, and strongly affirming your positive thoughts, will bring you to a new stage. You will learn to be emotionally literate—that is, to see and accept your true feelings without judgment or resistance. This stage also includes learning how to surrender and how to let go of control.

Other levels of self-knowledge will follow. You will learn to know your personal truths—that is, to become clear about what works for you and what doesn't, what you want and don't, or what feels right or good and what doesn't.

At this point, you will find yourself accepting all aspects of self without judgment, letting go of internal criticism, and engaging in loving self-practices.

The upshot of this process of self-strengthening is a trusting relationship with yourself that is the foundation for courage and risk taking. Now you are ready to express truth to the external world. You will do this not only by your ability to communicate personal truth to others, but also to set boundaries and to take risks to do new things so that your life feels vital to you and full of growth.

At this stage, you will find that life reflects the truth of who you are. Once you have achieved true awareness, you'll find that your everyday life will be full of positive changes, and with those changes there will arise in you the desire and willingness to experience more passion, energy, and enthusiasm for life and to express that new passion creatively.

## Personality Traits and Reclaiming Your Self

Everyone knows there are different parts to his or her personality. In order to start your own journey to self-discovery and total health, your mental, physical, emotional, spiritual, social, and intellectual personality traits should be evaluated to ensure balance in your life. Imagine for a moment, a pie cut into five slices that correspond to the major personality traits.

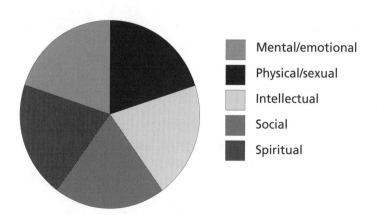

Let's say the five slices of the pie represent the following traits:

1. Mental/emotional
2. Physical/sexual
3. Intellectual
4. Social
5. Spiritual

Maximizing the potential of each trait helps ensure balance in your daily life. Equally important, each trait should work in harmony with the others and be as proportionate as possible. It is this integration of our personality traits that allows us to be happy and have the energy or motivation to accomplish our goals. If one trait is missing or not well developed, unhappiness and emotional fatigue can occur. Happiness and contentment become more prominent when your personality becomes more balanced.

Check each of the following statements that you feel is true about yourself.

**Mental/Emotional**

_____ I feel sad and dissatisfied most of the time.

_____ I regularly misplace and forget things.

_____ I cry easily.

_____ I feel angry or frequently resentful.

**Physical/Sexual**

_____ I don't wish to have sex because of the way I look.

_____ I am dissatisfied with the way my body looks.

_____ I have more than five pieces of clothing that I love and can't wear because they don't fit.

_____ I have had problems reaching a climax with a partner or by myself.

**Intellectual**

_____ I haven't read a book in more than six months.

_____ I wish I knew more about current events.

_____ I feel intellectually inferior to my spouse, partner, or mate.

_____ I wish I could go back to school.

## Social

_____ I feel that I should be more social.

_____ I wish I had more friends.

_____ It has it been more than six months since I went out to a social event.

_____ I feel more at ease when I am alone.

## Spiritual

_____ It has been more than six months since I've gone to church.

_____ I want to pray more.

_____ I wish I knew how to meditate.

_____ I wish that I deserved my Higher Power's love more.

_____ I have no Higher Power.

If you checked five or more items, see which category was checked the most. This is the trait you need to start working on.

Each of your important personality traits, when faced with stressors, can come under fire separately and affect the way you think and feel. Keep in mind that although I talk a great deal about regaining balance and becoming healthier by proper eating, food is not a part of our personality. This is the reason it is vital to discover what makes you tick from within in order to become healthier.

It's no joke that we settle into certain patterns of behavior that are detrimental to our health. Both my mother and Ms. Brown did, and I'm sure that some of you are doing the same. Individual habits, after all, are tied to ethnic traditions based on our cultural roots. Black-eyed peas and greens saturated with pork fat have long been staples of our diet. How do women of color change generations of attitudes and behaviors to develop healthier eating habits? How do they balance their personalities and integrate them to lose weight?

I can't express strongly enough that your journey toward better health starts by connecting with other women in a heart-to-heart way. A patient once told me, "Before I started connecting with women, I was depressed and my life was lacking a lot. My friend helped me remember my connection with other women and after a time I gained an inner strength and feelings of connectedness with everything around me. It basically healed my life."

Many of my patients have found support for embracing and taking control of their lives through other women and sister circles. Something powerful and magical happens in a community of women of color—something that helps you make sense of your world. Sharing with other women can help release the frustrations, hurts, and anxieties of life, and allows you to feel connected to the divine.

The decisions you make after reclaiming your self will leave you empowered to make decisions from a completely new place. All these acts will bring wholeness into your life and create a feeling of greater stability that enables you to take the risks necessary to create a life that fits the truth of who you are. Once your life begins to reflect who you really are, true joy, passion, and celebration can begin.

## *Three*

# WHY IS FAMILY MEDICINE SO IMPORTANT TO WOMEN'S HEALTH AND WEIGHT LOSS?

*We can all be angels to one another. We can choose to obey the small stirring within, the little whisper that says "Go, ask, reach out." Be an answer to someone's plea. You have a part to play, have faith. Wherever there is someone to help, the angels are watching.*
—Joan Wester

FAMILY MEDICINE PLAYS an integral role in African American culture. Historically, the family medicine model is rooted in tradition. It has helped many African Americans achieve maximum health for body and mind throughout many generations. In Africa, during ancient times, the medicine man and woman provided healing and social direction for members of the tribe. Today, the family doctor is still important for health guidance and care in the Black community.

Family medicine treats the whole person, which includes the impact that environment plays on a person's health. It treats the total family, yet pays very close attention to each person's individual needs. Today, family medicine is underused by millions of African Americans, not because it is lacking, but because people often don't understand what role the family doctor plays.

A family physician is, to put it simply, the Black woman's most important ally in becoming and staying healthy. Yet many African American women don't have a physician. Connecting emotionally with a culturally sensitive doctor whom you can trust is critical to your health and well-being.

As a strong Black woman, your needs are important and unique. But you may not find yourself always best served by agencies presumably designed to meet your needs. Do you use quick-service clinics or emergency rooms? If so, you probably don't receive the follow-up attention or care you need, and they probably ignore your emotional and cultural needs.

It's time to realize that the family physician is one of your best allies. A good family doctor is sensitive to your whole being and doesn't see you, or treat you, as simply a number. The family doctor provides the furthest thing from the quick-service approach that often leaves Black women feeling shortchanged and poorly understood. Let me illustrate with a story.

Marie is an eighty-five-year-old woman who acts and thinks like someone who is thirty-five years old. Her husband, Mel, the same age, is a retired army colonel. Neighbors of ours, Marie and Mel are a delight to be with. One evening at dinner, Marie, who is never without words, told us of recurring leg pains that had bothered her for some months. Her family doctor had recently retired, and so he referred her to one of his colleagues.

The new doctor, as Marie went on to tell us, "was this type of doctor who seemed to care less about what I was telling him and more about how many patients he should see. He ushered me out the door in five minutes and didn't tell me what I should have done about the pain." She went on to say, "The only thing he did was take his gold stethoscope and place it on my chest, pretending to listen to my heart. He didn't touch me or my legs."

Marie was adamant about telling the story to us. And she probably felt it important for me to hear it since she knew of my talks and books about sensitive family doctors and the care they give to patients. Marie, like many women, was appalled by the slapdash medicine of the doctor she visited. (A Harris poll, administered by Harvard University, showed that 60 percent of those with managed care insurance felt that their doctors did not spend enough time with them.)

Marie remembered how family doctors once were the confidants, friends, and protectors of their patients. She even told us that when she was a child, her family doctor delivered most of the children in her neighborhood and was always available for her family. She wished that these young modern doctors were like the doctors of old.

When Marie was sharing her story with me, I thought about the countless other Black women who felt the same way. Perhaps they, too, define family medicine by the doctors who have very little time for them. I want to dispel the myth that all family medicine is this way. The majority of family doctors are trained to practice with the care of the entire person in mind, and definitely do so.

Marie did not take her negative experience with this doctor passively. She made an appointment with another doctor right after her bad experience. When she told us about the second doctor, it was quite a different story.

"The new doctor was great! She listened to me, and unlike that other doctor, took a complete history. I don't think my old doctor of twenty years ever took such an intense interest in my health. I was able to tell this new physician things about myself that I never told another doctor because she took the time to listen. I told her of my fears of death and becoming weak and helpless, and that my husband had just had a mini-stroke. After this, the doctor gave me an exam from the top of my head to the tip of my toes. Can you believe she even felt my toes? In addition, she gave me an ultrasound to see if I had good circulation in my legs, and she said that she wanted to see me again in a week. What a good doctor! She is like those doctors I used to have."

The moral of the story is obvious enough. If you find yourself badly served by the kind of efficient but cold and uncaring medical treatment Marie received at the hands of her first doctor, seek out a family doctor who wants to give the human attention you need. All that's required of you is firm motivation.

A patient of mine, whom I'll call "Tina," shared a story with me about how she gains motivation. Tina is thirty-five years old, a professional woman with braids to her waist and an outgoing personality. She and her girlfriends have been getting their hair done at LaShawn's Hair Place for the last five years. She told me that she liked to call it her "sister circle" because while the women get their hair braided, they talk about everything under the sun, and the braiding process, which can take up to four to five hours, gives them plenty of time to "let their hair down."

Tina told me that during one evening, the subject of doctors came up. Aside from the banter about who had what ailment, they talked about their level of satisfaction with their healthcare. Remarkably, only two of the ten women in the sister circle were happy with their doctors, both of whom happened to be African American physicians and culturally sensitive to their needs. These doctors gave the two women the tools they needed to participate in their healthcare. The rest of Tina's friends had either foreign-trained or white doctors, and one of the girls—worst-case scenario—went to the emergency room for her primary care.

A good doctor–patient relationship is built on trust, regular communication, and a shared commitment to identifying goals and following through with care. The success of your relationship with a family doctor depends on a two-way commitment—rather than simply allowing the doctor to take charge.

Years of relating to patients have led me to understand that, as a Black woman, you are unique in many ways. Each of you presents to your physician a composite of many different personality traits. Along with your physical symptoms, you also display emotional symptoms. Family doctors are not simply listening to your physical symptoms; they are looking for the emotional clues as well. For example, if you visit your doctor because you have high blood pressure, you might want to share your emotional concerns as well so that the doctor can explore other possible causes of that high blood pressure.

A longtime patient of mine had been feeling overly tired for a year after her successful cancer radiation treatment. She had beaten the cancer, but her fatigue went far beyond the normal recovery period. This baffled the specialist she had been seeing. Upon further questioning about her personal life issues, I found that she had been overlooked for a job promotion after fifteen years with her company. To make matters worse, the person who got the promotion had less experience than she and was white.

Compounding her feelings of insecurity, my patient was required to attend a company lunch at a place that had historically excluded Blacks. The "invitation" reminded her of the painful issues surrounding her uncle who, years before, had been refused service at the very same restaurant because he was a man of color. My patient was understandably depressed and angry. It had adversely affected her daily life and, of course, her health.

A culturally insensitive physician would not have been able to pinpoint the real source of this woman's fatigue. Only her physical complaints would have been treated. In all likelihood, if I had not been sensitive to her dilemma, my patient probably would have kept silent and continued to suffer.

In another instance, a patient whom I'll call "Tanya" had recently gone through a bitter divorce and was searching for information about a community organization that could offer her emotional support. The first doctor she visited belonged to a health maintenance organization (HMO). He was from Southeast Asia. To her chagrin, even though he practiced medicine in her neighborhood, he had no clue about how to help her with community support, nor was he patient enough to try to understand what she was going through. "Why don't you see a psychologist?" was his only suggestion.

Sadly, Tanya left this doctor and went back to the urgent care center at the emergency room. A psychologist was not the long-term answer for her. As a new single mother, she needed community support to help her with childcare, financial matters, and spiritual guidance. Culturally sensitive family doctors are in tune with the needs of African American women and men.

Tameka, one of the women whom you'll meet in depth later in this book, is fifty-two years old and for three years has been treated for obesity and heartburn (heartburn is a term that is often used for gastritis or peptic ulcer disease) for three years. She, like many Black women, hated taking medicine for something that she felt God would cure for her. But every time she stopped taking her medicine, she would have pain in her stomach and gain weight.

Although Tameka wanted to enter the wellness program I was offering in my office, she told me that she had too much to do at home. During a family consultation, after I spoke with her husband about what was going on in her life, I began to understand her situation. Tameka, a very religious woman who took things heavily upon herself, was distraught that her son was lazy and had no desire to get a job. To make matters worse, her husband had just gone on disability for a bad back and was no longer working either. Tameka felt as though she carried the burden of her family on her shoulders. She internalized her negative feelings and used food to soothe them.

This is where I, as a family doctor, had to step in and explain Tameka's health issues to her family so they could understand how she was setting herself up for poor health and how they would need to play a part in her well-being.

Family doctors can do this for you. Urgent care physicians and emergency rooms are not equipped for this. If you don't already have a family doctor, it is time to find one to help you on the road to wellness. That means finding one who is sensitive to your cultural needs even though this isn't always easy. You need to be somewhat aggressive in the way you do it. Here are some suggestions on how to start:

1. Start making phone calls. The first should be to the National Medical Association, the major organization of African American doctors in America. The NMA has a program called NMA Physicians Locator Service. Call 888-662-7497 to find an African American physician in your area.
2. Ask your relatives, friends, and co-workers who their doctors are and what they like and dislike about them.
3. Call a doctor referral service at a local hospital. But keep in mind that these services usually refer you only to doctors who are on the staff of that hospital. They rarely give information on the quality of care that these doctors provide.
4. If you are enrolled in a health maintenance organization (HMO) or a preferred provider organization (PPO), call their customer service number and ask for a list of doctors in their health system. They may be able to tell you what criteria they use to select doctors for their health plans. They also may be able to identify a doctor who has the specific characteristics you need or prefer.
5. If you have a chronic health problem like hypertension, dia- betes, or asthma, you may need a doctor with a special expert-

ise. Contact the local chapter of the organization devoted to the problem, like the American Heart Association (for a cardiologist or heart specialist), the American Diabetes Association (for an internist), or the American Lung Association (for an asthma specialist), and ask if they make referrals.

6. Look in your local telephone directory, in the yellow pages, under "physicians." Advertisements or listings in these directories will help you identify doctors and the kind of medicine they practice. But remember that you cannot judge the quality of services from paid advertisements and directory listings.

7. Some local medical societies offer lists of doctors who are members. Check the yellow pages under "Associations." Again, these lists do not have information on the quality of care that these doctors provide.

It is also important that you know something about how the healthcare insurance system is set up. There are four types of health insurance:

1. Fee-for-service: You pay up to a certain amount for your health service and then your insurer pays for the rest.

2. Managed care: Your HMO pays for most of your care; however a co-payment may be required when you see the doctor. Some HMOs allow you to choose whom you see, but others assign you a physician. This is not the end of the world. Most HMOs will switch your care to another provider if you simply request it. In each state, there is an African American Medical Association that has a list of family doctors in your community. Chances are they participate in most HMO plans. Check Part Three of this book for locations in your state.

3. Medicare: This type of health plan is a federal plan for the elderly. The patient pays a premium and an annual deductible. If you are hospitalized, Medicare usually pays for everything.

4. Medicaid: Medicaid is for the dispossessed. About 10 percent of the American population rely on this form of healthcare. This program is federally funded, which means the federal government pays the doctor for your healthcare service.

No matter which service you use, be sure to choose a board-certified primary physician who practices family medicine. This means that the doctor has gone through a year as an intern in a family medicine residency program and three years of post-training. Doctors who are board certified have a desire to help you with short- and long-term healthcare goals. They are the gatekeepers who can help you access a health plan and guide you to complete your wellness journey.

The doctor–patient relationship need not be confrontational to have your needs met. Share your culture and concerns with your family doctor so that you both have an understanding about the type of care that you need. Then act on the new information that he or she gives you. Take the ball and run with it. Be proactive and try not to rethink the past. Looking back on past failures can cause depression and limit the energy you need to stay on track. Look ahead, but not too far. Take every day as the day that you will accomplish your goals.

Such a partnership with your doctor is the beginning of your personal journey toward physical and spiritual wellness. You'll rejoice to discover all the benefits that will enter your life when you take charge of your own health and well-being.

At that point, too, you can reap the benefits that the modern medical system has to offer. For instance, more women are now getting the necessary mammograms they need to prevent and treat breast cancer, more children are receiving vaccinations than in past decades, and more patients are getting heart medicines to lower cholesterol than in years past. All these benefits are open to those who have learned to work as partners with their doctors.

However, obesity remains a serious health problem for many Black women. The culturally sensitive program set forth in this book worked for the four women whose life stories you will read about, and it has worked for hundreds of other women who have since started their wellness journeys. It has worked because it takes into account all aspects of what being a Black woman means so that changes on the physical side reflect changes on the emotional, spiritual, social, and intellectual sides. The family doctor can start the ball rolling for you.

# Four

# EMOTIONAL FITNESS

*To appreciate beauty, and find the best in ourselves and others; to leave the world a bit better; to know that even one life has breathed easier because you have lived; this is to have succeeded.*
—*Ralph Waldo Emerson*

I N ORDER TO BE SUCCESSFUL in your journey toward total well-being, your intellectual self and your emotional self must be in harmony. This means that you must be fully aware of what you think and feel. Although life itself consists of a series of changes, sometimes smooth and orderly, sometimes unexpected, good emotional fitness enables you to deal with these life changes in a positive way.

In order to find a greater capacity for joy in living, you need to spend time improving your emotional fitness. When you do, your strength, skill, endurance, and energy will improve; your relationships with others will become healthier; and any emotional pain you may have will diminish rapidly. If you don't form the link between thinking and feeling, new behaviors, especially those related to good daily nutrition and regular exercise, are difficult to master. It's one thing to know you should eat healthily and increase your energy expenditure, but putting this thought into action can be very difficult.

The emotional part of your personality is perhaps the most important for total wellness. If you feel positive, chances are you'll act. Positive, goal-oriented feelings are the key to success in any endeavor. We all have been depressed, anxious, fearful, sleepless, mentally confused, disoriented, helpless, angry, enraged, emotionally distraught, socially isolated, disaffected, or immobilized at some point in our lives as a result of an overwhelmingly stressful event or a series of less stressful events. It's how we handle stressors like these that distinguishes emotionally fit people from those who are not.

You've certainly heard of people who can take on big new tasks without a mental warm-up. These are the same people who seem to succeed in everything that they do. But how do *you* get to that point? Here are five steps to get yourself started:

1. Take a truly honest personal inventory. Admit there are certain things you would like to change about yourself. Write them down to affirm those things so that you can visualize them.
2. Look closely at your environment and the people around you. Are the people supportive and loving, or draining you of your energy? What can you do to change their demand on your time or to make your days less chaotic? List both the positives and negatives so you have a running list of the good and bad. Focus on tackling each of the negative aspects so that it can be transferred to the positive column.
3. Focus on and tackle each issue, one at a time, knowing that solutions will not happen overnight.
4. Share your inventory with someone you can trust. Chances are that person will not only support you, but also share his or her own personal inventory as well. If there is no one in your life with whom you can do this, a trained psychologist can assist you.
5. Once you have visualized a goal, work each day, one step at a time, to fulfill that goal. It doesn't have to be a major step. Remember, little steps lead to big ones.

*Women who have achieved good emotional fitness are best able to succeed at a wellness program that involves weight loss because they are not bogged down by negative thoughts.* Further, because they are self-motivated, these women tend to persist regardless of the obstacles. They control their negative impulses.

You are no different from those women.

# THE MENTAL WARM-UP

Success through emotional fitness is based on a number of components, including a mental warm-up that involves coming to terms with your emotional self, choosing positive goals and achieving them, and understanding that change takes time and discipline. I should add that it also offers a good deal of energy and excitement.

Your journey to emotional fitness begins with a mental warm-up. Start by determining a clear course of action for each day. Choose realistic goals, based on your own circumstances and your energy level that day (in some cases, the mental warm-up itself can invigorate you).

Think of the warm-up as "pumping yourself up." Turn your attention to the exercise and eating patterns you will have all day. Leave all of your other cares and concerns at the door. Cultivating an attitude of respect and gratitude for that special time you will spend with yourself is akin to what the Japanese practice when they bow before they compete.

*An emotional warm-up begins with a few deep, calming breaths.* This breathing exercise can take place even before you get out of bed or after you start your day. Keeping your breathing relaxed and steady, recall the excitement you felt as a child when you were about to do something new and special. Form mental images that create heightened emotional energy.

What works as a mental image is different for everyone. When I ran college track, the day before a race I would envision myself at the starting line and then finishing first. No one else can choose your emotional goal for you. It depends on what makes you excited and happy. *You have to find what fires you up about taking care of yourself.* Imagine yourself succeeding at your goals; picture yourself winning, and feel how much you can gain from some positively directed energy.

A sports psychologist once told me about a simple practice he used to motivate his soccer players, and it's the perfect example of how to get your mind and body in sync with each other. Tie a small weighted object (like a paper clip) to an 8-inch length of thread or string. Let the object hang by the string, held by your thumb and first finger. Hold the string still, then look at it intently and begin to imagine that the paper clip is swinging back and forth, back and forth. Continue to imagine this, and watch what happens. Next, while the paper clip swings back and forth, imagine that it is going in a circle instead, and watch the results.

This test demonstrates the phenomenon of ideomotor action, which simply means that if you can imagine movement, then you can realize it in fact. If you settle into imagining yourself doing something, your physical self will respond.

*The best part about mental imaging is that there is no failure,* and you can do it anywhere—on the bus, subway, in the car, at work, while you're watching television, or even while grocery shopping. Another great advantage of personal mental imagining is that it's free. You don't have to take lessons to learn it. You already possess this talent. The main requirement of learning to become emotionally fit through imagining yourself doing it is to be totally relaxed while you practice it.

So many hours pass in our lifetime where we do not concentrate on beginnings and endings. Rather, we go through our days wondering what's going to happen next. People who are able to achieve success at weight loss are able to concentrate on beginnings as a positive action in their own right, not something that is overwhelming. These people are able to see clearly the results at the end and are patient throughout the process.

*During your process of becoming emotionally fit, you will meet people who teach you things.* Your doctor is one of your teachers; your friends can be your teachers as well. Along the way, you will meet other people striving for the very same things that you are, but you won't find them until you begin to concentrate on your own pathway. You may experience unconscious resistance to learning something new because of a belief that you must live your life your own way or because you feel that you could never accomplish something that someone else has been able to do. An honest examination of yourself may reveal a low self-concept, and the only way to climb out of that thought process is to acknowledge the success of others and to realize that you deserve the same successes.

Going to a gym is a perfect example of how you can start caring for yourself. People who go to a gym for the first time often feel resistant to lifting weights or aerobic exercise because they are unfamiliar with the exercises. Even though I had exercised throughout my life, I felt insecure when I started lifting weights. The truth is everyone has to start somewhere, and after some repetition and by asking questions, the language and techniques of exercise will become second nature to you.

But whether you start with the goal of a regular exercise program or choose some other starting place, the formula is the same. To create solutions, you must first come to terms with how you honestly feel about yourself. If you feel good about all—well, let's say most—aspects of yourself, then you are likely to take care of what you feel good about, namely, yourself.

A young driver loves his jalopy and cleans and polishes it everyday because he does love it. He spends a great deal of time on that car. You deserve the gleam that comes from polishing your physical, mental, emotional, spiritual, and intellectual self.

As a Black woman, you work especially hard at taking care of others. You are often the backbone and the sacrificial lamb of your family. Working hard will get you a paycheck, but it won't make you healthier unless you're a trainer at a gym or health spa. We have been socialized into thinking money will make us happy, but if we're not healthy then it means little to be wealthy.

All too often, women develop the spiritual, intellectual, and at some level, social aspects of their personalities without concentrating on the physical and emotional aspects. You will see, however, that many of us exist day to day, ignoring needs that hinder us from achieving the happiness and quality of life and health we deserve. Focusing on the emotional part of your personality is important when you make a decision to become healthier and lose weight. It is invaluable for achieving health and happiness in your life.

## THE BENEFITS OF EMOTIONAL HEALTH

Today we understand more and more clearly that a person's physical and emotional health are tightly twined together. Stress itself, which can cause any number of health problems, can also contribute to obesity. Let me tell you a little about handling stress (see section three for tips on how to meditate and to do exercises that will help you with that job), and how to start your weight loss program without letting occasional plateaus or setbacks discourage you.

### *Handling Stress*

Emotional health defines how well we react to the stress in our lives. When faced with an emotional situation, there are several ways we can react. The key to a strong and healthy emotional component is to know the healthiest way to react to emotional situations, and through impulse control, to define that reaction by making it work for you.

If a person who is depressed, angry, or even psychotic from continued stress reacts impulsively, the emotional part of his or her personality suffers. So does his or her body. Such negative changes can also cause deterioration of the personality. You've seen such wounded persons—sometimes they seem like ghosts, sometimes they seem like demons.

You can see then, why we must learn to manage stress, and why doing that requires us to take responsibility for our emotions. Those two goals underlie everything else this book has to teach you.

### *Emotions and Weight Loss*

Emotional fitness determines how self-motivated women who participate in weight loss programs can succeed. The ability to persist when faced with obstacles is another factor. It is not how many times you get knocked down to the canvas, but how many times you're able to get back up on your feet that matters most.

Women who participate in weight loss programs have periods when they don't lose weight or when family members may try to tempt them to abandon their goals. But emotionally fit women can keep going and are able to maintain their strength when they hit roadblocks. Through emotional fitness, your self-motivation will increase. By making yourself your number-one priority, you will become self-motivated.

What happens as a result of emotional fitness is that you will eventually want to exercise and not see it as a chore. You will begin to make time for yourself during your hectic schedule to eat healthier and to be happy. Setting small daily goals and accomplishing them will cause you to become even more motivated to achieve more the next day. No one will have to tell you that planning meals is good for you. You will do it because you love yourself.

### Controlling Your Impulse to Eat Unhealthily

Controlling your impulse to eat unhealthily is another component of emotional fitness. It's something that can be learned. The women you will read about shortly worked hard to control their impulsive eating, but once they got past the first week, it became easier and easier. Here are some tips they learned to increase their emotional fitness and focus on impulse control:

1. Eat in a tranquil setting. In this type of environment, you will eat more slowly and pace yourself, placing the fork down while you chew your food.
2. Don't eat when you are upset or angry. Anger causes you to eat too much and binge.
3. Always sit down at a table when you eat. Never eat on the run or in the car.
4. Drink water, not sodas, and drink every fifteen minutes while you eat. This aids in better digestion of food.
5. Don't watch TV or read while you're eating. Never carry on a heated or serious conversation while you eat. This will cause you to overeat.
6. Place less food on your fork and finish chewing and swallowing all the food in your mouth before picking up the fork again.
7. Try to enjoy what you eat. Don't simply eat to be eating. Make eating a passionate ritual.
8. Sit a few minutes after you eat before moving on to something else. Try to clear your mind.
9. Try to vary the food you eat so that you don't get bored.
10. Eat to live, don't live to eat. When you snack, substitute fruits and vegetables for sugar-filled fixes.
11. Carry a card that says, "Stick with the plan!" Keep it with you

always, and if you feel compelled to overeat, read it out loud three times to reaffirm that you are following a plan that will have a positive outcome, and by sticking with it you will accomplish something that is yours personally.

Let me review the main points I've made. Emotional health helps you in many ways, everyday. It:

- Defines how you react to stress.
- Helps determine your self-motivation.
- Controls your impulse to eat unhealthily.
- Helps you control and delay gratification.
- Increases your self-awareness.
- Allows you to focus on the positive.
- Enables you to achieve happiness.

## TAKE IT SLOW BUT TAKE IT

The last component of emotional fitness is the ability to delay gratification. This important ingredient is very similar to impulse control but is long term and goal oriented. It's obvious that you didn't gain weight overnight, and you will not lose it that way either. It will take time and you must acknowledge that. Understand that if you take little steps toward your goal, the end result will be more rewarding.

Let me illustrate by sharing a story of my own. I started medical school at the age of thirty-five. I received little or no encouragement. People thought it was a silly idea for me to get a medical degree at my age because I would not become a doctor until I was well into my forties. But those people didn't understand that in my mind I already saw myself as a physician. That's what kept me forging ahead. And that same ability to move steadily toward a goal is what I want to share with you.

Keep in mind that the foundation for reaching your goals is self-awareness. Self-awareness starts to blossom when you become more aware of your moods and your thoughts about those moods. Even if sadness and despair are at the forefront of your emotions, you will quickly alleviate those feelings in a healthy manner instead of becoming stuck with them.

Just as important as managing bad feelings is the new happiness you will experience. You will learn how to change distress to positive outcomes. Women who know how to do this accept what they can't change, and change what they can. That balance is delicate. I once heard a story about a 5' 6" man who successfully willed himself to be 5' 11".

## INTRODUCING FOUR WOMEN

Let me introduce you to four women who met at the eight-week wellness program explained in this book. Each woman learned to acknowledge her negative moods and to talk about them before these moods defined her. That way, each woman was able to dissipate her negative energy quickly. In each other, these women found the seeds of vital emotional connection.

One of the women had a husband who didn't emotionally support her during the program. She had been very dependent on him for approval most of her life, and the fact that she wasn't getting emotional support made staying on track very difficult. She felt sadness at first. But the members of her support team helped her see that though she could not change her husband's attitude, she could get the support she needed from the group itself. She accepted this and was able to meet her wellness goals, calling the other women when she had a problem with her husband.

Another of the women had a boyfriend who had cheated on her in the past. Although they had reconciled, she felt he would cheat again. Her depression from past events blocked her from reaching her future goals. Her support team and I told her not to delve too much into the past; that what was done was done. She had to move on and not feel so insecure about what her boyfriend would do next. As a result of her involvement in our program, this woman learned to handle her feelings without looking back and to concentrate on her present goals. She learned not to depend on her boyfriend but on values more solid, and she, too, did well in the program.

Relationships are very important to women of color. Though relationships can sometimes bring pain, you treasure the love expressed by those you hold dear to your heart. Although love may seem an impractical thing, one way to preserve it in your relationships is by managing your time better.

Compartmentalize the things that are important to you by taking care of yourself first. Most people complain that they have very little time for exercise and activities like meditation. That's because people don't manage their time well. Our four women became proficient in making schedules, giving them time to do what they needed for themselves as well as for those they loved.

*All the women made their daily schedules out the night before.* They got up early so that they became masters of their days. Control of their daily activities allowed them to stay steps ahead, and adherence to their schedules became their own priority.

What these four women had achieved in four weeks are the same qualities you can realize in your life. It may seem like a dream list now, but you'll be surprised how quickly it can become real. As a result of emotional fitness, you will:

1. Become more assertive in reaching your goals and dealing with others
2. Be able to express your feelings more directly
3. Feel more positive about yourself
4. Have more meaning in your life
5. Become more outgoing and gregarious
6. Express your feelings more appropriately
7. Adapt to stress better
8. Be more playful and humorous
9. Become more spontaneous
10. Feel less guilty and anxious about your behavior
11. Feel more sensual
12. Feel more optimistic
13. Become more altruistic
14. Learn how to better soothe yourself

## EMOTIONAL FITNESS AND OBESITY

The American Medical Association defines medical obesity as being 30 percent or more above your ideal body weight. One popular method used to calculate obesity is the Body Mass Index (BMI). The BMI is a mathematical equation that tells how much body fat a person has based on his or her weight and height. The equation is as follows:

Weight in kilograms, divided by your height measured in meters squared

To figure your BMI, use the following formula:

1. Multiply your weight in pounds by .45 to get kilograms.
2. Convert your height to inches.
3. Multiply your height in inches by .0254 to get meters.
4. Multiply that number, your height in meters, by itself.
5. Divide your weight in kilograms by your height in meters squared.

For example: You weigh 200 pounds and are 5' 5":

1. Multiply 200 X .45 = 90 (this is your weight in kilograms).
2. Convert your height to inches: 5 feet X 12 = 60" + 5" = 65 inches.
3. Multiply your height in inches by .0254: 65 X .0254 = 1.651.
4. Multiply that answer by itself: 1.651 X 1.651 = 2.725 (this is your height in meters squared).
5. Divide 90 by 2.725 = 33.09

If your BMI is between 22 and 25, you're in pretty good shape and are deemed healthy with low overall risk. You are considered overweight if your BMI falls between 25 and 30, and you are considered obese if your BMI is over 30.

Everyone who participated in the wellness program in this book had a starting BMI of over 40. A large percentage of the African American women who have asked me to help them lose weight have been obese in terms of their BMI although not all of them were unhealthy in terms of their lab results.

Obesity is a growing epidemic that threatens the health and quality of life of millions of Black women in the United States. It does not discriminate between young and old. Even some elementary school girls are extremely overweight. That fact is alarming because research shows that overweight children are likely to end up as obese adults who have severe health consequences early in their lives, suffering from diseases like coronary heart disease, diabetes, and even cancer.

Today, Americans in general consume high-fat, high-calorie foods indiscriminately. They also exercise less. The result is that more and more people are becoming unhealthy and overweight.

In the *Journal of the American Medical Association* (October 27, 1999), the Center for Disease Control and Prevention stated that obesity in the American population increased from 12 percent in 1991 to approximately 18 percent in 1998, a 50 percent increase! And being overweight and not engaging in physical activity accounts for more than 300,000 premature deaths each year in the United States.

It's tragic. Our quality of life depends on how well we take care of ourselves. That is why *I wish so deeply for Black women to rediscover that they are the pinnacles of beauty, not the bearers of poor health.* Approaching weight loss from a "whole person" perspective will empower you to take control of your health and well-being, and so change your life.

All too often we say we'll start to do something sooner or later, but later just isn't soon enough. My sisters, now is the time to focus on the present, to start your journey to combat obesity and its health effects. It's time to become emotionally healthy so that your life can be full of happiness and wellness, so that you can do all the things you want to do throughout your life, so that you can live life fully and as life is meant to be lived.

# Five

# HEALTH LITERACY AND MOTIVATION

*My doctor really acts surprised every time my blood pressure shows*
*up normal, which is every time. And every session she says I should*
*lose weight. She says it nicely, but still says it.*
—Monica Persson

TAKING RESPONSIBILITY for your health and well-being does require much of you, but it requires something of your doctor, too. I've often heard doctors tell women to lose weight so that they can manage heart disease or diabetes better, or so that they will simply feel together. But unless the doctor also provides tools and support, he or she is simply telling these women that they are unhealthy.

Wellness and weight loss occur only when the doctor can provide tools and support to go along with the prescription. Sometimes there's a lot of resistance from the patient. Being told that you are obese can feel like a blow to your self-esteem, and if that's the way you take it, you may not have the confidence to act.

So let's get something straight right now: *you are in no way flawed as a result of carrying too much weight.* Wellness is not about appearances; rather, it's about taking care of your whole person and being able to do something because you want, and are able, to do it.

# WHY THE WORD DIET MAKES US FEEL SO BAD?

The word *diet* strikes a negative chord with nearly everyone. It's not pleasant to think that you might have to give up something pleasurable in order to lose weight. If I slip and use the word *diet* instead of *wellness* when I talk to my patients, they act as if I am taking away something very near and dear to them. That something is food. The word *wellness* means total health, but *diet* implies only two things: eating less food and becoming thinner.

Most people who have struggled with fluctuations in their weight have tried to lose it using various strategies, only to have failed in the long run. It is because of this association with failure that I stopped using the word *diet* to motivate and treat my patients. Ideally, "diet" should imply the broad range of food and drink that we consume every day for our survival—not the removal of food from our plates or weight from our hips.

Simple removal of food from our plates does nothing to help us become healthier. Sure, it might help you lose a few pounds in the short run, but in the long run, "diet" feels like a synonym for "deprivation."

Further, the word tends to make people think that there's a cause and effect action: if they eat less, they will lose weight. This couldn't be further from the truth. The result is that they feel defeated and depressed. The real story is this. When you do not eat, your body reverts to starvation mode, and it will actually overcompensate for the decrease in calorie intake by *holding on* to the calories that it receives. This is a survival defense mechanism that protects the body from harm. Not only does your body's metabolism slow down when you diet, but the stored fat in your body burns off more slowly. The result is that you don't lose weight, and when you again start eating the foods you have deprived yourself of, you will gain weight twice as fast.

# NUTRITIONAL ANSWERS YOU NEED TO KNOW

What is health literacy? Being "health literate" means that before you start any kind of healthy change, you understand what is going to happen to your body and how you may feel differently as a result of the program. Knowing these basics in advance and being aware of them as the changes occur will help make you successful. Health literacy means knowing how nutrients derived from the food you eat behave in your body, and how your metabolism (the speed at which your body uses nutrients) changes as a result of different food choices.

When I was training for a bodybuilding contest, I noticed that the gym groupies had a language of their own. The more I learned this language, the better my understanding became. It is the same for people changing their eating patterns. Learning makes you more capable, more efficient.

Believe it or not, many doctors don't know much about the importance of good nutrition in achieving and maintaining good health. That most laypeople know even less goes without saying. So here's a short course in the language of nutrition.

### Carbohydrates

Dietary carbohydrates are an important source of energy for humans. They include simple sugars and complex carbohydrates. Simple sugars are small molecules that are responsible for the sweet taste in food. Complex carbohydrates are not as sweet, and consist of long chains of sugars that can be found in starches such as potatoes and corn. The body uses carbohydrates by converting them to glucose for energy. Glucose is the preferred fuel molecule for the brain.

Also composed of sugar are fibers. Although the body does not absorb fiber, fiber serves as a significant aid to digestion.

Almost all carbohydrates are derived from plant foods. Some examples of simple sugars are candy, cake, cookies, donuts, ice cream, and fruits. Aside from fruits and fruit juices, the other examples contain very small amounts of nutrients and should be limited in a healthy diet. Some examples of complex carbohydrates are breads, cereals, crackers, pasta, grains, rice, vegetables, and beans. They are nutrient-rich foods because they contain vitamins and minerals. Many of them also contain fiber.

### How Our Bodies Use Carbohydrates

As the body digests carbohydrates, it stores the converted glucose in the liver except for what is used immediately for energy. There, the glucose converts to glycogen. During the first few minutes of exercise, glucose is the primary fuel. However, after about twenty minutes, the body starts burning the stored glycogen. Fat burning follows. About 70 percent of the body's fuel comes from glycogen; the rest comes from fat. That's one reason exercise is so important. It burns fat.

### What About Protein?

Protein is crucial to our body's organs. Fibrous proteins are the major components of muscles as well as of skin, bones, tendons, blood vessels, teeth, and hair. Blood contains proteins responsible for the storage and transport of biologically important substances such as oxygen, glucose, and fats, as well as many other molecules. Furthermore, proteins called enzymes participate in all the different chemical reactions that occur in the body to break down the foods we eat and generate energy from our diet.

Proteins are involved in the transmission of nerve impulses, and they play a significant role in our thought process and movement. They also protect the body's immune system.

It is possible to use protein for energy, but that is one of its least important roles. Only during starvation does protein become a direct energy source. If protein is not replaced through a healthy diet, body tissue will break down. Since the body can't store extra protein as it can carbohydrates, you must eat adequate amounts of protein to ensure that your body gets enough, especially during weight loss.

It is important to eat enough protein to prevent the loss of muscle mass. The normal daily protein requirement for women is about 50 to 85 grams a day, but for our program the women were placed on high-protein regimens, closer to 100 grams of protein a day. (Later in the book, you'll see how these numbers translate to the actual food on your plate.)

Some scientists believe that higher amounts of protein may be bad for your kidneys though current research has not shown this unequivocally. Nonetheless, to be safe, I strongly recommend to all of my patients that they increase water intake to flush the system. As I will discuss later, it is also important that, before you start on a wellness program, you take a blood test that shows kidney function.

Foods with high protein value should make up at least 15 to 20 percent of a woman's daily calories. Lean meat, poultry, or fish can provide this. Egg whites are an excellent source of protein and make a good meat substitute. Each ounce of animal protein contains about 7 grams of protein, each dairy product about 8 grams of protein, and each complex carbohydrate about 3 grams of protein. Vegetables contain about 2 grams of protein per serving. Protein drinks, which you can buy at nutritional stores and supermarkets, often have 30 grams or more of protein per serving.

### Tell Me About Fat

Fats can be complicated because it is hard to keep all the terms straight—which are the good fats—saturated or unsaturated or monounsaturated or polyunsaturated?

Fats are organic compounds made up of carbon, hydrogen, and oxygen; they are the most concentrated source of energy in foods. Fats belong to a group of substances called lipids. Fats come in liquid or solid form. All fats are combinations of saturated and unsaturated fatty acids. Fats can be called very saturated or very unsaturated depending on their proportions.

The word *saturated* here means that a particular fatty acid is saturated with hydrogen atoms. We have found such fats bad for you because the high amount of hydrogen makes it harder to dissolve in the body.

The body needs fat in order to function. Fat is one of the three nutrients, along with protein and carbohydrates, that supply energy to the body. Fat provides 9 calories per gram, more than twice the number provided by carbohydrates or protein.

Fat also provides the "essential" fatty acids, which are not made by the body and must be obtained from food. Blood pressure is controlled by the raw materials produced by fatty acids in the body. These same materials also control blood clotting, inflammation, and other body functions.

The role of fat in the body is storage of extra calories. Fat deposited in fat cells helps insulate the body. When the body has used up the calories from carbohydrates, it begins to depend on calories from fat.

Healthy skin and hair are maintained by fat. Fat also helps transport the fat-soluble vitamins, A, D, E, and K, through the bloodstream.

In addition to providing energy, fat helps maintain cell and tissue structure, cushions the body's internal organs, and protects them from trauma. Finally, if it weren't for fat, we would have to eat constantly to meet our energy needs.

Having said all that, I must add that too much fat hurts the body in a variety of ways that we are only beginning to map.

### Saturated and Unsaturated Fats

Saturated fats are usually solid at room temperature. Some foods that contain high levels of saturated fats are stick butter and margarine, meat fat, bacon grease, egg yolk, chocolate, cold cuts, hot dogs, sausage, and cheese. Whole and lowfat milk, coconut, and palm oils are highly saturated. *Make sure you read the number of grams of saturated fat on labels.* A good strategy is to read the labels on several brands of a food you intend to buy. If one has 30 grams of fat and the other has 25 grams of fat, then common sense would have you choose the lesser fat content.

Remember, saturated fat calories should not exceed one third of the fat calories and 10 percent of the total calories per serving. It is also important to understand that *saturated fats are most responsible for raising blood cholesterol and laying down plaque in the arteries, which leads to coronary artery disease.*

Monounsaturated fats are liquid at room temperature. Monounsaturated fats have been associated with lowering blood cholesterol levels. Examples of foods that are high in monounsaturated fats are corn, safflower, sesame, soybean, and sunflower oils; tub margarine; and fatty fish such as salmon, herring, whitefish, and sardines.

### *About Cholesterol*

Your blood cholesterol levels should be below 200. Cholesterol is often contained in foods that are also high in saturated fat. Cholesterol intake should not exceed 200 mg daily. Cholesterol is a waxy substance and can build up in the arteries, forming hardened plaque that diminishes and blocks blood flow. The result can be a heart attack or stroke.

Cholesterol is contained only in animal foods because it a byproduct of, and is manufactured in, the liver. High-cholesterol foods are liver and other organ meats, whole milk, cheese, beef, pork, veal, egg yolks, and shrimp.

### *What Are Triglycerides?*

Most body fat occurs as triglycerides and is carried through the blood attached to small particles called lipoproteins. Lipoproteins are labeled according to their density.

LDL means low-density lipoproteins, HDL refers to high-density lipoproteins, and VLDL refers to very low-density lipoproteins. LDLs and VLDLs are harmful and can cause blockage in arteries.

Triglycerides are a source of energy, too. But high levels of triglycerides increase the risk of heart disease and are associated with diabetes, obesity, alcohol, and sugar consumption. Butter, margarine, and oils are dietary sources of triglycerides. Triglyceride levels should ideally be below 150.

HDLs, or high-density lipoproteins, are the helpful type of cholesterol that can protect against heart disease. HDLs are the "good" guys because they remove excess cholesterol from the arteries. High levels of HDL are good for you. Low levels are caused by smoking, obesity, and lack of exercise.

*High HDLs come from a healthy diet and exercise.* Omega-3 fatty acids contained in fish have been associated with decreased cardiac risk because these fatty acids lower blood cholesterol and triglyceride levels, and slow the rate at which blood clots, thereby reducing the chance of heart attack or stroke.

## Nutritional Myths About Weight Loss

To achieve wellness and lose weight, you need to know the truth behind some common myths that might derail your journey. So let's review some of those myths now.

### Myth 1: The Less I Eat, the More Weight I Will Lose

When I started practicing medicine, I thought patients were not telling me the truth when they said that they ate only one meal a day and still could not lose weight. However, after many years of studying nutrition, exercise, and body metabolism, I now know that they were being truthful.

*To burn off fat, you need to eat more quality calories,* which means you can really eat a great deal of food, but certain kinds. Steamed and baked vegetables, small portions of broiled or baked lean meat, turkey and chicken, soy products, and fresh fruit are all examples of the kinds of foods that can be eaten in abundance.

Meals should not be large; eat small portions and have healthy snacks in between. At first, you need to count calories so that you know exactly how much you eat per meal. After a while, counting calories becomes second nature, and you begin to look at food for its nutritional energy value rather than impulsively eating something simply because it looks good.

For example, if you take in 1500 calories a day, and eat five meals a day, divide 5 into 1500 and you get 300; 300 calories per meal and five or six of these meals a day would be ideal.

If you schedule more frequent healthy meals throughout the day, each with fewer calories, your body becomes thermogenic, or "hot." The warmer your body is, the faster you burn fat. Eating a small meal every four or five hours will increase your metabolism, and balance your body chemistry so that you burn off more fat.

It's the same principle as placing more logs on a fire: the more logs, the bigger the fire. Our bodies work the same way. The more efficiently you feed it, the more resourcefully it burns off energy and the more weight you lose. So don't consider this a book about losing weight or dieting. Rather, it is a book about achieving overall wellness.

*Myth 2: If I Drink Water, I Will Hold onto Water and Gain Weight*
How many times have you heard someone say, "I don't drink water because I hold water terribly." The body is made up of approximately 80 percent water. So whether you do or don't drink it, the body will hang on to what it has. Wouldn't *you* if you were being deprived of the one nutrient that keeps you alive? The truth is drinking more and more water will actually help speed up your metabolism and acts as a diuretic so that you lose water.

Further, when you change your eating patterns to eat healthier, you will increase the amount of protein in your diet. Therefore, it is important that you drink water to flush your digestive system. Some people who retain water do so because of the high salt or sodium content of their diet; others have problems with their kidneys that can also cause water retention.

A simple adjustment in daily eating habits, such as implementing a low-sodium diet, can reverse this water retention. If you do experience serious fluid retention, it is important that you let your doctor know. The recommended daily intake of water is 64 ounces per day (eight 8-ounce glasses).

*Myth 3: Carbohydrates Are Better Than Protein*
Whether carbohydrates are better for you than proteins depends on whom you talk to or what books you read. One author made a fortune proposing a carbohydrate diet. The friendly pizza boy will tell you that his doughy pizza will give you energy and is good for you. Carbohydrate loading, a recent fad, probably did more "harm" than good, even for the athletes who advocate "carbohydrate loading." Studies now show that carb loading does not increase an athlete's energy stores or increase his or her chance of winning.

Although carbohydrates do give you energy, they should never be the biggest part of your diet. Why not? Let's say that you eat two slices of bread for breakfast, three slices of pizza for lunch, a plateful of mashed potatoes for dinner, and ice cream for dessert. You watch a little TV and then go to bed. The problem is you have not used up all the starch and sugars, which are what carbohydrates are, during the time you sleep. That bread and ice cream turns into fat, and that's no fun. The result is that you have to increase daily activity to burn off the excess carbohydrates you consume.

One of the biggest health problems for many Americans is that we consume too many carbohydrates and not enough protein. Personally, I think that the American diet is protein deficient, and that's why diseases like obesity and diabetes have increased this last millennium. Protein is needed to burn off fat because the more muscle you have, the more energy is needed to sustain it. Where do you get that muscle? From exercise, of course! This energy is taken from carbohydrates stored in the body. Instead of excess energy stored as fat, energy is transferred to keep muscle strong.

### Myth 4: If I Take Vitamins, I Will Get Fat

Vitamins don't make you fat; eating too many carbohydrates and not burning them off makes you fat. Yet many women believe the vitamin myth, and it's so hard to change their minds about what vitamins do and don't do.

Vitamins are enzymes that make things happen. They take the nutrients like fats, carbohydrates, and proteins that we eat and help deliver them throughout the body. Without them, your body becomes as inefficient as an engine that is badly in need of oil. Imagine for a moment that you're in a subway station waiting to go someplace. You look around and you see many other people on the platform also waiting for the train. Finally, the train arrives and transports all the people to their respective destinations. In this example, the train performs like a vitamin or enzyme, and the people are the nutrients.

Vitamins are usually needed only if your diet is not as healthy as it should be. Many of my patients don't eat enough leafy green vegetables. Because of this, it's important that they take vitamins with folic acid and other B nutrients. Vitamins provide that source without making you fat.

### Myth 5: If I Eat Meat, I Will Gain Weight

Meat does not necessarily make you fat. If you eat chicken, fish, turkey, and very lean beef, you can enjoy it. Meat contains protein, and protein is the building block of muscle. Meat can be lean, with a very low fat content, or high in fat. The key is to select meats low in fat.

Meat is not converted into fat unless you eat meat products high in fat. Meat products are made up of amino acids that produce the muscle in the body. The more muscle you have, the more you'll burn off fat. Since I have used the term *muscle* a lot, let me say just a few words about it.

If you eat more protein and do exercises using light weights, you will not grow the muscles of a bodybuilder. This is another myth that women have. Instead, when you change diet patterns and add exercise, you recompose your body by refining the percentage of fat on your body and adding more muscle. In essence, you become more toned.

In addition, the more protein you eat, the less water you retain. Carbohydrates act like sponges and hold onto water, whereas for every gram of protein you eat, you lose 9 grams of water from your body. By the way, protein helps brain cells grow; therefore, protein is called brain food.

### Myth 6: All Fat Is Created Equal

I've said this once, but it's so important that I'll say it twice: *all fat is not created equal.* Monounsaturated, polyunsaturated, and saturated fats are different. Saturated fat is the worst for you. Saturated fat can clog arteries, thicken the blood, and when eaten in abundance over long periods of time, cause heart attacks and even stroke.

Monounsaturated fat is the best for you. Olive oil is an example of a food product that contains monounsaturated fat. Polyunsaturated fat falls in the middle between saturated and monounsaturated. Always try to read food labels to determine what type of fat a particular food contains.

### Myth 7: I Don't Have Time to Exercise

Not having enough time is a myth. In a society of conveniences, we tend to blame everything on a lack of time. The fact is if you don't find time to take good care of yourself, then you will actually lose time in your life. Those people who take the time to care for themselves live longer and healthier lives. They are also likely to be more productive.

If we love ourselves the way we should, we must make time for ourselves. Make time for quiet meditation so that you can find your spiritual self, and make time for exercise and other ways to find wellness.

*Part Two*

# SISTERHOOD CONNECTIONS: THE JOURNEY

# Six

## Four Women

*I don't know how much I weigh these days, though I can make a good guess. For years I'd known that number, sometimes within a quarter pound, known how it changed from day to day and hour to hour. I want to weigh myself now; I lean toward the scale in the next room, imagine standing there, lining up the balance. But I don't do it. Going this long, starting to break the scale's spell, it's like waking up suddenly sober.*
—Sallie Tisdale, in A Weight That Women Carry: The Compulsion to Diet in a Starved Culture

THE ADDICTIVE FERVOR ASSOCIATED with getting thinner is everywhere. You read it in the headlines of a newspaper, on magazine covers at the supermarket, or some billboard along the road that touts "thin is in." The diet hoopla is unfair because it sends negative messages to women that they are not worthy of any indulgence if they do not look like the air-brushed models represented in the media.

Of course, the fad is profitable. There are thousands of books on the shelves that tell you how to exercise and get fit, but many are so confusing that it's not even worth the time it takes to read them. There are even fad diets, with catchy names like "sugar busters" or "the watermelon diet."

By focusing on the newest ways to lose weight, and attempting them, we set ourselves up for failure because, quite frankly, they simply do not work. Sure, perhaps you lose weight in the short term, but that's where the yo-yo dieting comes into play. Over many years, many women and men who attempt to lose weight, just give up because they are not geared for long-term success.

*When it comes to losing weight, it is all about changing your lifestyle.* This doesn't mean you have to change the way you do everything, but you have to be aware of the dynamics of your life in order to make a successful change. Some people have long-term success by changing on their own, but most people who attempt to change deep-formed facets of their lives need help.

The program we're giving you in this book is successful because it focuses both on you the individual and on your active sense of community through sisterhood. *Your* work is to reconnect with your individual self and to figure out what makes you tick. As to sisterhood, because people who change need help, you'll best reach your goals if you work with a group of women who also want to change. In such a group, each member becomes a key support to every other member.

As you well know, community and social connections are the cornerstone of African American roots. Women of color are, by nature, expressive. You support each other in good and tough times alike, and unlike many Black men, you understand that this connection is an important part of accomplishing your goals in life. So forming a support group will feel natural to you.

To sum up, a program of change based on the "sisterhood" principle works better for Black women than does an individual weight loss plan. The four women you are about to meet participated in a wellness program that emphasized collective emotional support and relied on group goals for weight loss. The four women certainly didn't come out of the same experiences, but each woman's life had been riddled with obstacles and disappointment. Some had wealth and others did not, but together they all gripped tightly to a common goal, and that was to get healthier together.

I'm sure you will identify with some of the complex issues they faced while on our wellness journey. And if you do what they did during the eight weeks they were using this program, you also will experience the same success! These are real women, real stories.

# MEET TAWANDA

Tawanda was a twenty-year-old college student who was working her way through college. She had supported herself from the age of seventeen because she wanted to be independent. She worked purely from her need to feel independent. Her father had been absent from her life since she was three, and her mother, with whom she was very close, died of a heart attack at the age of forty-two when Tawanda was just thirteen.

In part because her mother had been a schoolteacher, Tawanda had always been a high achiever in public school. She knew the importance of getting an education and was determined to finish school with honors. But when her mother died, Tawanda found herself overeating a great deal, admittedly for comfort. She would snack all day and overeat at meals.

At thirteen, her weight was normal, but during the four years she lived with her aunt, Tawanda gained a great deal of weight and acquired terrible eating habits. What got her in trouble weren't only her own impulses to soothe her grief with food. Her aunt believed in always keeping enough food in the house to feed everyone who stopped by, and there were no real-time constraints on when they ate, which is what led to Tawanda's way of snacking all day and late into the evening.

Tawanda received an academic scholarship to the University of Pennsylvania. After one semester, she wanted to get her own place to live and to get a job, even while she continued in college. She didn't like living with others in a dormitory.

But the new stress of both going to college and working to pay rent took its toll on Tawanda's body. At twenty years old, her weight was over 270 pounds, on a frame just 5' 6" tall. Tawanda naturally became more and more self-conscious and defensive about her appearance.

When Tawanda originally came to see me, prior to starting her quest to lose weight, she confided that she became winded when she walked upstairs, could not keep up when bike riding with friends, and was basically tired all day. The weight was contributing to her depressed moods, and she told me that even going to the doctor's office was a chore.

It became evident to me after talking with her for a while that she really resented the way doctors had treated her in the past. She was defensive from the start, even before seeing the doctors, because getting up onto the examining table was difficult and being asked to change into a small gown that showed her backside was embarrassing to her. As a result of this humiliation, she stopped going for regular medical care and told me that she had taken a chance even seeing me. I could tell she was not used to asking for help.

After careful consideration of Tawanda's past, and after talking with her a great deal, I concluded that she was, first and foremost, depressed. I referred her to a psychologist who began treatment. After approximately six months of therapy, Tawanda came back so that I could help her lose weight. I wasn't certain she was ready because she was still dealing with some issues of loss relating to her mother and she was not accustomed to working with a group, but I agreed to begin treating her.

During the first couple of weeks in the group, Tawanda broke all the rules. She did not drink the eight glasses of water a day that everyone was instructed to do, and she cheated relentlessly on Tastycakes (a Philadelphia favorite) because it was an easy snack between classes.

She also had some resistance to increasing her daily activity by taking stairs instead of elevators, but she managed to summon up the energy to accomplish this.

As reluctant as Tawanda was to changing the way she'd always done things, she slowly became more optimistic because others who were in the program with her were encouraging her. Also helpful was that one of the women in the group, precisely at 6:00 a.m. and without fail, knocked on Tawanda's door every morning to wake her for their morning walk. It was a blessing that both women lived in the same neighborhood. This prevented Tawanda from isolating herself from the rest of the group.

Early in Tawanda's life, she had been encouraged by her mother to participate in sports. Her mother had been very conscious of her daughter's health, and she herself had played softball and basketball with her friends. With her mother's death, Tawanda had retreated inside herself and withdrew from sports because the activity reminded her so much of her mother.

What she didn't realize was that she could keep those wonderful memories alive by continuing in sports and by opening up to others. This was one of the points we tried to reinforce during our group meetings over the eight weeks. Tawanda did not have to be alone any longer.

One of the more poignant reasons that Tawanda wanted to lose weight was that she didn't want to die like her mother. She, like her mother, had been diagnosed at an early age with a congenital heart condition, which is what had caused her mother's untimely death. If Tawanda did not take control of her eating habits and start exercising, it was likely that she, too, would be at risk for the same fate.

Consequently, Tawanda realized the seriousness of the situation. Getting started was the hardest part for her because change was scary. However, during the course of her therapy with the psychologist, Tawanda began to recognize that by taking care of herself, she would also be memorializing her mother. It was, after all, her mother who had taught Tawanda to take care of herself by exercising and eating well.

She could still use her mother's guidance to take control of the many things that caused her emotional pain. But now, little by little, Tawanda let the group help take the place of her mother. She began to talk to the others about her daily activities and eventually opened up her emotional life to everyone else. She even talked about her half-hearted attempt to end her life several years ago and how hopefulness had replaced the despair she once felt.

The next several chapters describe in detail how Tawanda came to better manage her time, walk regularly, eat more healthy foods, connect emotionally with others, and take control of the events that caused her pain.

Tawanda lost 35 pounds during the course of eight weeks.

## MEET DIANE

Diane is a thirty-five-year-old Black woman who, unlike Tawanda, had a happy and cheerful disposition. She was more outgoing and did not dwell on things or brood too much. Like Tawanda, Diane didn't like being alone either. Her personal motto, "woman can't live on bread alone, she needs meat and potatoes," made us laugh, but held a considerable amount of truth about how Diane lived her life. She never looked back on past mistakes, didn't dwell on things that had no relevance to the present, and was happiest when she was eating and socializing with family members and friends.

Raised in a religious family, Diane was taught early on that God wants people to help the lonely and the despondent. She was a nurturer and had a motherly quality. Therefore, it didn't surprise me that she was drawn to Tawanda.

Diane is 5' tall and weighed 265 pounds at the start of the program. She did not really understand how serious a condition her weight was and how changing her eating habits could affect her ability to continue to help people. But all that was about to change.

Diane's family life had been cohesive and supportive. Her mother was a homemaker and her father a popular local minister for a large church congregation. Diane worked as the church's administrative secretary for many years, and had started fresh out of high school. Her talent for organization and writing would have enabled her to work almost anywhere that required administrative skills, but she chose to remain at the church because of her deep faith in God and because it allowed her to work closely with other people in the congregation. In short, she wanted to do God's work and to do it through a community.

Genuinely satisfied to stay at a place where she grew up and where everyone knew and liked her made change exceedingly difficult for Diane. Moving toward a new approach to life was going to require more effort from her than from the other women in the program because Diane was basically happy with her life the way it was.

As a child, because Diane was always larger than the rest of her peers, her parents, also obese, never encouraged her to take gym or to exercise. She said in her first group meeting that her family was like the Klumps in the movie *The Nutty Professor*, where everyone in the family was fat, and it was the norm. She naively added, "We're just like them for the most part. We are happy and we eat well. The best time we have together is dinnertime."

She reminisced about the big dinners her family always had. "Black folks," she claimed, "had a culture that was centered around the dinner table and that's where the most wonderful gatherings were." She had a good point, but I thought Diane wasn't seeing the total picture. She didn't take into consideration the health consequences of years of hearty eating. Her family celebrations led her to eat whatever she wanted, whenever she wanted, whether or not it was healthy for her. Consequently, she had equated being "happy" with eating food.

But Diane's early avoidance of exercise in school was something she was uncomfortable with. She told me, "My father always wrote letters to the school nurse to excuse me from gym. The excuses said I had asthma. Don't get me wrong, I did have asthma, but not as seriously as the notes to the school indicated. I suppose my dad was trying to help me."

Sure, Diane's size and her not exercising made other kids tease her, but she had good self-esteem, and the biting remarks from classmates didn't bother her. Once, in fifth grade, the school nurse told Diane she had to go on a diet. But when Diane told her parents, they ignored the nurse's instructions and even brought ice cream for her that same day so she wouldn't feel bad about what the nurse had said.

Church events didn't help either because all the activities seemed centered on food and praise. Diane said that many church members were large and carried a lot of weight. I began to wonder why Diane had made the decision to be a part of the group and lose weight in the first place. I would soon get the answer.

Diane was serious about a young man for the first time in her life. He told her that he was in love with her and asked her to marry him, but because of her weight he was worried about her health. At that point, Diane began to connect her body with her health. Because she still lived with her parents and might perhaps get married and move, she wanted to be the very best companion she could possibly be for her soon-to-be husband. This decision in itself was a healthy start for her.

Diane's father and mother were happy for their daughter, but at the same time sad that she would not be living with them anymore. But throughout the program, it was Tawanda, interestingly, who always intervened with quiet encouragement, telling Diane that by losing weight she would not only be healthier for her new husband, but for her parents, too.

Most important, Diane would be better for herself.

A person's motivational style affects his or her ability to move toward healthy eating and exercise habits. Diane is an extroverted person. She is outgoing, motivated by the end result of achieving positive goals. Tawanda, on the other hand, is much less outgoing and more guarded; she is introverted. End results tend not to be effective motivators for an introvert. Following rules and ultimately getting a reward are better motivators for this type of person.

So Diane's path would be a path of achievement. The health and happiness she would experience by losing weight and exercising will give her the opportunity to help others. That would be her motivation. Tawanda, on the other hand, finds more success following a directed course of action. Her reward would be her reconnection with her mother's early encouragement in her life.

At the onset of our program, Diane had high blood pressure and elevated cholesterol levels. Because we had talked about everyone's physical conditions during the initial meeting and physical, she decided that her first goal would be to bring these risk factors into a normal range.

Diane had never exercised or played any sports, so over the eight weeks, members of the group helped her with these. Since Diane's good humor and spirituality were intact, and her social nature was magnetic, she would prove to be a great role model for the social and spiritual aspects of the program, and would eventually be motivated by helping others achieve this sound and spiritual growth.

Diane, as you will see, did not readily accept the facts about obesity. What changed her was looking at her situation from the perspective of being able to help others. If she were well and healthy, she would be able to continue doing what she loved most: making other people happy.

During the course of the eight-week program, Diane lost 36 pounds.

## MEET ROSE

I had the unique pleasure of meeting Rose when she was hospitalized for abdominal surgery a few years ago. She had just had her appendix removed and was looking for a family physician. During my rounds at the hospital, I recall that her young children, who lived with their father in Florida, were with her in the room. Neither they nor I could know that our relationship would soon be about something even deeper than abdominal surgery.

Rose is a thirty-seven-year-old pharmacy technician. Standing 5' 3", she weighed 250 pounds. Rose is very intelligent and has a pleasant disposition. Adopted at birth by adoring parents, she was showered with love and affection throughout her life. Her adoptive parents gave her the best gift of all, an educated view of the world. Rose's father was a chemist, her mother a nurse. Raised to believe she could accomplish anything she set her mind to, she set out early on to get her degree at a Louisiana university.

Rose grew up concerned about health issues because her adoptive mother was obese, had diabetes, and later died from the disease. Rose had cared for her mother during the last few years of her life. She witnessed an assortment of ailments in her mother that resulted in hospitalizations, the amputation of her legs, and a focus for all the family on homecare. Experiencing the debilitating effects of diabetes in her mother helped Rose see the importance of wellness.

Rose found in me a doctor who shared her interest in fitness and nutrition. It wasn't that she hadn't looked for one earlier. But most doctors, she said, were insensitive to her rapid weight gain, and often they themselves were overweight. Her doctors simply didn't seem to have much knowledge about the causes, the implications, and the effective treatment of obesity. Even doctors who claimed to be all about prevention, focused on her symptoms and not necessarily on why she was having trouble controlling her eating and exercise habits. I saw that Rose's insight would bring much to the group, so I invited her to join us, and she accepted.

Rose had graduated with honors from a local university one year prior to her entry into the wellness program. Employed by a local pharmacy chain, she studied during her free time with the goal of going to medical school. She felt by joining a wellness program, she would be able to regain her focus on herself, as well as make herself stronger mentally and emotionally in her quest to become a doctor. Losing the large amount of weight she had accumulated over the past few years was just the challenge she needed.

Rose's life was complicated. She had been an honor student in high school, but her precocious behavior got her into trouble at home. She went to wild parties and experimented for a time with drugs and alcohol. Despite all that, she maintained an A average in her coursework and later enrolled at Louisiana State University. But after a year, she dropped out to pursue a life of fun and travel.

After moving to Florida, she married a jazz musician and had two children, a boy and a girl. Unfortunately, her husband was an emotionally abusive man who neglected Rose. She never went back to college and settled into a life of stress, poor eating, and confining her life to the domestic role in her relationship.

Despite the trouble in her marriage, Rose became a successful hairdresser and eventually started her own business. Then this, too, became a strain on her marriage because her husband thought she was spending too much time away from home. Rose sold the business and went back to taking care of the family.

All through this her father stuck by Rose and hoped that one day she would finish college and do what she really wanted to do— become a doctor. His steady support no doubt helped Rose finally see that she was not in a healthy relationship. She started taking steps to get a divorce.

During her years of being unhappy, trapped in an endless loop of disappointment, Rose became extremely overweight. She had gained so much weight that she stayed in the house and away from people. Losing confidence in her abilities, over time she had ballooned to nearly 300 pounds. That is when she decided it was time to find someone to help her. A doctor she went to suggested that she join a gym.

Of course, Rose's husband wasn't happy about her decision to change and reclaim herself. He tried to sabotage her plans by making more and more demands on her time. Rose even said that he would leave the young children alone, so she was forced to stay at home. He resented her newfound motivation and belittled her when she returned from the gym. "You'll never be anything more than a hairdresser," he had said. That's when she snapped—and began to see the light.

Although time management had been a problem for her, Rose began to get up at 5 o'clock, before anyone else in the family, to go to the gym. She made meals for herself aside from those she prepared for her family. After more than a year of dedicated workouts, she lost close to 150 pounds. She regained confidence and control over her life.

By that time her marriage was basically over and her husband, who continued to be nonsupportive, started cheating on her. But Rose kept on. It was during this time that she set a goal of entering a bodybuilding show. The next year, she did so, and proudly took third place in a bodybuilding contest in Florida. Rose's story was very powerful for everyone else to hear, and it made me proud that she was to be a part of the program.

Little did Rose know, however, that her biggest obstacle lay ahead: the divorce itself. Rose took the children and left her husband. But because she was dependent on him, she was ill equipped financially to fight the custody battle that ensued. She was strapped because she had no way of paying for a good attorney, and her husband had hired one of the best divorce lawyers in the city. Sadly, she was forced to leave her children behind with a man who lied to the courts about her ability to care for them.

In the months following, Rose met a professional man who only wanted the best for her. Although it was probably one of the hardest things she had ever done, she moved away from her children, to the Philadelphia area, to reclaim her life, which included going back to college.

When I met her, Rose was totally preoccupied with getting her kids back. She completed college with honors even though she had gained almost 100 pounds again. She jumped at the chance to join the group. Having more knowledge about exercise and nutrition than the others did not distance her from them. On the contrary, she became an asset to everyone. Because of her past weight training, athletics, and knowledge of exercise, she was a mentor to us all, including me.

Rose also advocated women participating in sports because she felt women of color still remained a minority in the sports arena. One of the biggest issues that she often thought about was how outdoor recreation was nearly nonexistent in many of her friend's households and in the neighborhood where she lived. Her primary goal for the group was to help reduce the myth that Black women simply don't exercise.

During our program, Rose lost a whopping 41 pounds over the eight-week period.

## MEET TAMEKA

Tameka is a fifty-two-year-old lawyer whom I was treating for stomach pain, ultimately diagnosed as ulcer disease. I had known her for two years prior to her entrance into the program. She had always expressed her desire to lose weight, but her attempts to follow a prescribed nutritional plan and exercise regime had always failed because of her lack of discipline when it came to food. Tameka made no secret of the fact that food gave her a warm feeling inside and that she loved to eat. At 231 pounds and 5' 5" tall, she was on a path toward poor health and a limited quality of life if she didn't do something now.

As a busy law partner in a large firm, Tameka knew the importance of follow-through, but had trouble applying it to her own life. When presented with the opportunity to have support while trying to get healthy, she anxiously joined the group simply because she was afraid to fail again.

After high school, Tameka had married an older man, and they had opened a restaurant in the inner city where she cooked and managed the business. She was an artful chef and soon had many customers who traveled miles just to taste her food. Everything went well for many years. Money was no problem, and Tameka became a mother of a young son.

One frightful evening, a night that Tameka tries to forget, her world came to a crashing halt, and she was terribly unprepared to deal with the aftermath. Two hooded men came into the restaurant and tried to rob her. While trying to negotiate with the gunmen, her husband was shot and killed. Tameka suffered emotionally for many years until she finally found a psychologist who helped her through the turbulent coming to terms with her husband's death. After several years of therapy, she was finally able to move on with her life.

Tameka stayed a single parent for several years. During that time, she sold the restaurant and started law school. She met a man who became her constant companion, and they married soon after she finished law school. But bad luck was on her side again. Her new husband had a stroke and became disabled, needing constant care and attention. Tameka's son, now a teenager, had developed a drug problem. Tameka began to feel drained and powerless.

After working long hours during the day at the law firm she was now a partner of, Tameka would come home to care for her bedridden husband and make sure that her son didn't steal anything from the house to sell for drugs. Ultimately, she became seriously overweight and developed an ulcer from all the stress.

From his sickbed, Tameka's husband argued with her about the way she treated her son. He thought she was too hard on him and blamed her for his drug use. The stroke had made him angry and irritable, and nearly impossible to live with. Tameka began to resent both of them.

Like Diane, Tameka was religious. Her strong faith in God prevented her from leaving her family. She felt it was her responsibility to take care of both of them, and make things work just the way they were. As long as Tameka took her medicine, she did not have stomach pain. She did everything for the family and sacrificed most of her own needs. Like most women in her position, exercise and healthy eating habits were not a part of her lifestyle, nor even a priority. Feeling helpless to implement a change in her own life, she explained to me that she was just too busy doing everything for everybody else.

Reluctant to enlist in the wellness program because she was older, insecure, and she thought, too pressed for time to commit to an eight-week program, Tameka gave up before she began. But after contacting her several times, and being politely told no during each phone call, I told her during my final call the date and time of the first meeting. To my pleasant surprise, Tameka showed up for the first meeting and stayed for the entire program. Tameka paired up with Rose after realizing that they had the same hairdresser in common. They were good for each other and for the group.

With my help, Rose volunteered to take charge of the exercise part of the program.

Tameka was the food expert, not because she knew the nutritional value of the foods, but because she wanted to learn. Her creative background and cooking experience from her early days as a restaurant owner proved to be an asset. She helped with meal selections and variety. During the eight weeks, Tameka learned to become a better time manager of her personal life.

She lost 31 pounds during the program.

Here are the goals I gave to the four women prior to their starting the journey:

- Begin to think about the way you eat and drink. Pay close attention to your eating habits and what it is that you eat.
- Try thinking about how comfortable you will be asserting yourself. Try to put yourself first at least once prior to the first meeting. Remember, first and foremost, you're the most important person.
- Stop one bad habit (for example, snacking or eating big meals late at night).
- Take time out to relax each day. Buy a book on relaxation and meditation. Read at least ten pages a week during the eight weeks.
- Make a list of ways to decrease stress in your life and discuss them with the group.
- Begin to think realistically about what you can accomplish from week to week and try not to concentrate on the entire eight weeks.
- Write down all the positive things that will occur as a result of the program.

What's extraordinary about our wellness journey is that the women worked together toward a common goal, and as you'll see, they succeeded.

## THE FOUR WOMEN IN A NUTSHELL

### *Tawanda*

Biggest issue: Depression and mood swings
Best trait: Open to help

Personality trait most dominant: Co-dependency
Best asset: Good athlete
Biggest obstacle: Resistant thinking
Final weight loss: 35 pounds


### *Diane*

Biggest issue: Time; wants to lose weight before wedding
Best trait: Spiritually grounded and happy
Personality trait most dominant: Self-satisfaction
Best asset: A desire to help others
Biggest obstacle: No knowledge of nutrition or exercise
Health dilemma: High blood pressure and high cholesterol
Final weight loss: 36 pounds


### *Rose*

Biggest issue: Emotional eating
Best trait: Easily motivated
Personality trait most dominant: History of acting on impulse
Best asset: Excellent knowledge of exercise and nutrition; natural
     teacher
Biggest obstacle: Wants to get into medical school
Final weight loss: 41 pounds


### *Tameka*

Best trait: Spiritual and organized
Best asset: Great cook; knows success
Personality trait most dominant: Tendency to put needs of others
     before her own
Biggest obstacle: Time
Health dilemma: Has ulcer disease
Biggest life issue: Son on drugs and invalid husband
Final weight loss: 31 pounds

# *Seven*

# WEEK ONE

TAWANDA, DIANE, TAMEKA, AND ROSE all arrived at my office on a Tuesday evening at 7 o'clock sharp. We met in my conference room, where I had fruit and a vegetable tray with nonfat dip waiting for them, along with diet sodas and tea. I put together a packet of healthy eating brochures from the American Heart Association and slipped in a notebook and pen for their record keeping and journals. Each woman greeted me at the door then made a B-line to the food and health literature. While I watched them introduce themselves to one another, I smiled because I have always admired the way women are able to connect so quickly.

Black women are not caught up in the competition and posturing that Black males (perhaps most males) incline toward. Ego simply does not get in the way of common goals. This is why women of color embrace their female role models with open arms.

Before the first meeting, I had given each woman a complete physical exam, which included laboratory blood testing for diabetes, heart disease, high blood pressure, thyroid and metabolic disorders. All four women signed a patient consent form agreeing to participate in the eight-week wellness program. Even though each of them had other medical conditions that I was monitoring, their blood tests and physical exams showed they were healthy enough to begin.

During that first meeting, all the women weighed in. Tawanda weighed 270 pounds, Diane was 265 pounds, Rose weighed 250 pounds, and Tameka was 231 pounds. Each was considered by medical standards to be obese using Body Mass Index (BMI) measurements, but that didn't seem to bother them because now they were motivated and on their way to wellness.

The chairs were arranged in a circle, and as the four found their seats, I shared my happiness that they had all made it and arrived on time, sensing that was a good start. They were attentive, enthusiastic, and serious about our new wellness journey. I informed them that the theme for the eight weeks was "Love."

I said to them, "This is a love journey, which means that you will learn how to love yourself better during the course of the program. You will become healthier and lose weight at the same time. The eight-week program will meet once a week on Tuesday evening at 7:00. Each of you will keep a journal on what you do and eat during this period. The journal will also allow you to write down feelings, both good and bad, that you will have during the eight weeks. It may be tough at first to write everything down, especially when some of you are not accustomed to writing down your feelings and behaviors on paper. But don't despair; you'll get used to it as time goes on."

I told them I would provide them with suggested foods and exercises to choose from, but I also made it clear that as time went by each of them would probably develop her own eating and exercise plans.

"Each week we will pick a topic to discuss. The subjects could range from nutrition to exercise to personality and emotional issues. In fact, our meetings will, in some aspects, resemble a support group where we might end up talking about anything and everything without fear of embarrassment.

"Each of you is here to help the others and to be available for emotional support whenever there's a need. That's what community is all about. Don't be shy about bringing your thoughts to the discussion. Whatever is said here stays here.

"Since this is a journey of connecting with each other for a common goal, we will work together in pairs. You will each have a partner, but this doesn't mean that you cannot connect with the others. During the week when we're not here meeting, each of you will call or schedule a time to meet with your partner to discuss progress or possible problems that may come up. You will all have each other's phone numbers, including my home phone."

None of the women had known each other before that night, but it was evident that it didn't matter because they were chatting up a storm and realized that they all knew someone that the others knew. The brief time at the snack table gave them ample opportunity to know who would be whose partner.

Rose said, "Can we pick now?"

"Sure," I said.

Tawanda and Diane picked each other, which left Rose and Tameka paired. For some reason, this didn't surprise me. Tawanda was more reserved and inclined to stay to herself. She is quiet most of the time and not very animated. On the other hand, Diane is very outgoing and always happy and cracking jokes. Opposites did attract.

Tameka and Rose, on the other hand, were much more alike. Both were very intelligent and academically oriented. Rose was mature and wanted to be a doctor. Tameka was older, settled, and a lawyer. Both women shared a dominant personality, and they seemed to integrate very well with each other.

In my mind, it didn't really matter what type of personality any of these women had as long they were willing to work with another whatever her background might be. If the collective goals were the same, the individual goals would be accomplished without much friction.

As our discussion moved forward, I asked each of the women to share why she wanted to participate in the wellness program. Tawanda said to everyone emphatically, but without much expression, "When Dr. Smith told me that he was going to do this wellness group with other women, I knew that I had to get involved. It seemed like the time to lose weight and finally get myself together. I just went through a bad period with my boyfriend and decided that I needed to start taking better care of myself. When my mother was alive she used to encourage me to exercise. Since she died, I haven't really been motivated. Losing my mother was the worst thing that's ever happened to me and it's been tough." She reluctantly went on,

"Most of the time I feel down and tired, so this program is ideal for me to try something new and get a fresh start. I think by working with other women who have the same goal as me that I'll be able to get outside of my own head."

"Praise the Lord, everybody!" exclaimed Diane. "When God gives you a sign that it's time, it's time. I'm happy to be here and I don't really know anything about diet or exercise. I came here because I think that the group can help me lose a little of this," Diane said as she pointed to her belly. Everyone giggled along with Diane as she continued, "The doctor's been tryin' to get me to lose weight for a long time. I just haven't been able to do it. At first I wanted to do it because I have someone else in my life besides God; a new man, thank you very much. But, I was just talking to Tawanda before we sat down, and we both started talking about our boyfriends. She said, 'Girl, you need to do this for yourself, not that man.' I know she's right and I'm ready to stop listening to his telling me how fat I am, and get healthier for me. There's a lot of people out there I want to help and I need all the energy I can get. The pounds can't be around," she laughed. "Praise the Lord!"

Diane put her hands down after singing her short praises, and Rose piped up. "I want to love myself more and get back on the track that I was on before I stopped thinking about myself first. I used to train constantly in the gym and always lifted weights. I even entered a bodybuilding contest before and came in second place. But, you would never know it by looking at me. I feel really bad about it. What have hurt me along the way have been nasty custody disputes that I've had with my ex for several years. Each time I get going good, he throws a wrench at my moods. I study, too, so it's been tough. If it's okay, the doctor said that maybe I could help the group with dumbbell exercises, and it might help me feel better again."

"Rose, I'm gonna take you up on that dumbbell thing," said Tameka with a shake of her head and a little attitude in her voice. "I've always wanted to give that a try, but going into the gym really isn't for me. I just can't stand the fact that all those skinny little people would be looking at me. Also, I work so hard at home and on my job that I seem to have very little time for myself. Something's got to give. I have a son that's driving me crazy 'cuz all he does is lay on the couch, and a husband that I have contemplated getting rid of, so I'm ready for this.

"Yes, Diane, I think God wants me to get a grip on myself. My biggest problem is finding time for myself. I guess when it comes to taking care of me, I'm a poor organizer of time. Dr. Smith said that this is a wellness program that shows you how to take care of yourself first. Maybe the diet and nutrition will be good for my stomach problems, too."

All four women seemed open and willing to freely share information about themselves. They talked a great deal, which surprised me, because up to now I knew that I was the only one whom they'd told their stories to, and I wasn't sure if they would be this open this quickly. Although the program had a strong emphasis on motivation and techniques that would strengthen each area of their personalities, I was happy to see that each woman seem to be very excited about being here and appeared to be motivated to start a new life's journey.

After everyone got to know each other a little, we took a break and returned to the introduction of the program: reviewing the importance of good nutrition throughout the eight weeks. I wanted especially to talk about how to recognize protein, carbohydrates, and fats in their diets. "Okay, it's time to take out your notebooks," I said. "The three major nutrients are protein, carbohydrates, and fats. And water is important, too." I then talked about what these nutrients did and why they were important.

"Protein aids in the development of tissues and cells," I started. "For example, protein helps muscle to grow and skin and hair cells to become more beautiful." When I said that hair, skin, and nails would grow and become healthier, Diane yelled out, "That's what I'm talkin' about," and all the women started laughing.

Once the laughter died down, we went on discussing protein. "Scientists," I said, "are aware of the importance of protein and use it in the form of enzymes and antibodies to fight disease. In addition, protein is being used, in some instances, to treat the debilitating disease Alzheimer's. Increasing the protein in your diet will also help burn off fat and provide a source of energy once the sugar in your diet decreases. This is because when you eat more protein, you build muscle."

I reassured all of them that *they would not grow big muscles but become more toned* in the process of exercising. "Since the energy it takes to sustain muscle is greater than the energy your body requires to hold onto fat, the energy used first is the stored fat.

"But how do I tell the difference?" Tameka asked, confused.

Rose then said, "It's all different kinds of meat, chicken, turkey, eggs, and fish. Really, if you think about it, everything else is a carbohydrate."

Sitting back listening to Rose and Tameka talk made me realize that this is what the program needed to be about: women helping women.

"So, anything that clucks, moos, or swims?" Diane said jokingly and with a chuckle.

Rose said, "Yep, you've got it!"

Knowing that their conversation would be a nice opening to talking about carbohydrates, I said, "We're all carbohydrate junkies. There's something about sugar, potatoes, and pasta that all of us can relate to."

"But I don't eat a lot of cookies and junk food," Tawanda replied.

"Well, it isn't really the actual junk food that makes us gain weight. Rather, it's the amount of carbohydrates we eat versus the amount we exercise. What happens is that the sugars and starches we eat become stored in our bodies as fat," I said slowly.

Tawanda scratched her head and looked up and then exclaimed, "So, all I have to do is cut down on that and get moving again, and everything should really come together?"

"Well, it's not that simple, but close. You have to make good food choices, and the junk food has to be eaten in careful moderation!" said Rose with a smile. "My biggest problem is those carbohydrates, too. There's nothing like a big plate of spaghetti."

"My carbohydrate of choice then," said Diane, "is a king-size Snicker's bar."

Laughing again, Tameka said, "Pie, pie...oh how I love pie!"

With a smile, I said to the women, "Okay, I'll reveal my biggest carbohydrate fixation, it's cheesecake." Needless to say, everyone shook her head in agreement. "But I have a great no-sugar, lowfat recipe for cheesecake, so you can actually eat it during this program."

One of my goals was to give all the women a good foundation in macronutrients, and increase their sensitivity to exactly what sugars and starches were, and how they acted in their bodies. I told them, "Don't get me wrong. We need carbohydrates as our main source of energy, so you should never cut them out altogether. Nor do I advocate seriously low-carbohydrate diets because you can experience low blood sugar. The type of carbohydrates you eat and the concentration of it in each of your meals is important for good health. If, for starters, you maintain a 50 to 60 percent carbohydrate concentration per meal, you'll be safe."

Since I knew that only Rose was a real water drinker, I made drinking water the next nutrient that I reviewed. Diane was resistant to the idea of drinking eight glasses of water a day, and turned up her nose when I mentioned they needed to drink as much water as they could. "Just carry a personal water bottle around with you, wherever you go. It might feel strange at first, but keeping track of how much water you drink will ultimately help you to be successful in your diet. If you don't drink enough water, you will have problems eliminating the increased protein and fiber you will be eating. If you don't drink enough water, you will become bloated, and feel more uncomfortable and fatigued during the course of the day. Constipation is a common problem for people who don't drink enough water," I said.

"Oh is *that* what causes that?" Diane said mischievously. Again, the room erupted in laughter.

"Let's move along to the evil culprit of weight gain. Fat in our diets," I said. "Fats are needed for energy and for cell structure. They are also important for the hormones that women need."

Rose asked, "What about this omega-3 fat that I hear about? Isn't that supposed to be a good thing?"

"Yes, omega-3 fatty acid helps the body put on muscle and helps to prevent certain types of diseases. Some studies have reported that omega-3 fats can help decrease heart disease and certain types of cancers. These fats are found in fish," I said. Then I noticed that Diane had a wrinkled brow. I looked at her and told her, "Don't worry, by the time you're done, you'll know exactly what the nutrients are and just what they do in our bodies."

I suggested that everyone try, during the first week, to limit their intake of fat and to pay close attention to food labels. Since this information was new to everyone but Rose, I only wanted them to start thinking about the amount of fat they ate and cooked with. I recommended they use unsaturated fats or nonfat substitutes, and asked them to keep track of their fat intake by writing down in their journals how much they ate.

After a quick break, we started a discussion about motivation because Tawanda was worried that she couldn't motivate herself. I told them about my own experience while training for a bodybuilding contest. I showed them my before and after pictures and blushed as each of them made cooing noises and laughed. I let them know that if it weren't for the support of my wife and others, I might have had a problem with motivation, too. "Because this group is all about supporting one another, you will have each other and me to draw motivation from," I said emphatically.

"It's no secret that many people find it difficult to get up early and exercise on their own. Without someone encouraging you, you have to rely on something deep inside of yourself to push you. You all have it inside of yourselves, but finding it might take a little while, so don't get discouraged," I told them.

The women agreed they would work as a team. They all felt that their chances of success were better because they had each other to rely on. When one member of the group felt a little lazy, another would be the motivator. Any problems could be addressed individually with one another or brought to the group for discussion. By talking and sharing thoughts, everyone would be able to draw on a pool of broad experience.

"The way we'll do this," I started, "is that each of you will take turns being the group leader for that week. Then, you'll alternate. The leader will take the initiative to check on her partner, and make sure that she sticks to what it is she is supposed to do to maintain her effort to reach her goal. Taking on this responsibility will motivate the team leaders to do the same. The team leader, for example, could be the alarm clock and wake her partner if they agree to get up early and exercise. Or if one of you needed help with planning a meal, then the leader would be there to help with suggestions."

Toward the end of the meeting, I instructed the women to take a multivitamin with calcium. Tameka, at that point, questioned whether or not vitamins would make her fat. This is a common myth embraced by many women of color. "Vitamins don't make us fat, Tameka, eating too much does," I explained. I told them that the calcium was needed to build strong bones, which they needed because part of their journey involved exercise and resistance training with dumbbells. Building strong bones and preventing diseases like osteoporosis is important for all women.

The next topic discussed at this first meeting was the number of calories to eat and the suggested number of meals per day. "I gave you notebooks to keep journals on what you eat and how much you eat. In terms of calories, I would like you to eat 1500 to 2100 calories a day. It is important to divide the total number of calories *by the five or six meals you'll eat each day.* By this calculation, you come up with approximately *350 to 400 calories per meal.* In order to stick to this number of calories per meal, *you absolutely must start to read labels,*" I said. Then, pulling out a can of soup and a box of cereal, I pointed out that the Food and Drug Administration (FDA) required companies to put on their food labels how much protein, carbohydrate, fat, and sodium was in a product. The food label was going to be their guide when making food choices.

"Sodium," I said, "is the same as salt. Most of us know that people with high blood pressure should reduce their salt intake. However, even people with normal blood pressure may benefit from less salt in the diet, especially if they are salt sensitive. *Studies have shown that many Blacks are salt sensitive, and eating too much sodium increases their blood pressure.* Each of you will have no more than 1000 milligrams of salt a day.

"The first thing that will happen as a result of limiting your sodium intake is that you will actually lose excess water, making you feel less bloated. Many African Americans are salt sensitive and as a result retain water. This is why the doctor gives you a diuretic."

At about this point, Tameka said, "Fine, but let's get down to it. How do we get rid of the fat we've already got?"

"To burn off unwanted pounds by burning off fat," I told the four women, "you will eat several small meals a day. This will allow you to feel satisfied, and it will keep your blood sugar levels normal so you won't get tired or mentally dull. When metabolism speeds up, you'll also burn more fat. One of your meals will be a nutritional snack."

"You mean, like potato chips?" Diane asked, deadpan.

"No, not sugar snacks, but something healthy, like a power or nutrition bar or a protein drink. Some of these can be purchased at a health food store, and they don't cost an arm or a leg. This means that I would like all of you to start cutting the simple sugars in your foods. The cakes and cookies have to go. But it's okay if you want to buy some of the diet sweets that are sold at your supermarkets. Try to drink diet sodas also, and don't worry if you don't like the taste at first because you'll get used to it. When down the line you can eat a sweet treat from time to time, it will be a wonderful sensation."

When I started to talk about walking for exercise, Diane rolled her eyes as if to say, "Oh no, I knew it." Neither Diane nor Tameka were enthusiastic even a little about the idea of structured exercise, but I assured them that once they made it a part of their daily routine, this feeling would change. I suggested that when they drove to work, they park farther from their building. The longer walk would be good for them, body and soul.

I also mentioned that taking the stairs instead of the elevator was a great idea. Walking around the block in the early morning hours when the sun comes up is also a perfect way to start the day. "I would like each of you to start off slowly at first so that you can build up as time goes on. Walking even at slow and measured paces will help you speed up your metabolism and burn off calories. If you want to increase the intensity of walking this week, it would be okay, but start slowly so that you don't get discouraged," I said.

I had covered a lot for our first meeting, and I didn't want to overwhelm the women. As we broke up, I stressed that by starting the program off slow, they were more likely to feel better. As the weeks went on, they would be better able to assess what worked for them and what did not.

During this first meeting, Diane, Rose, Tameka, and Tawanda were all given the emotional inventory that can be found in Part Three of this book. They were instructed to take it home and answer the questions, and to bring it back to discuss during next week's meeting. The inventory would give the women an idea of what they needed to address from an emotional standpoint to keep them from becoming stuck. Emotional stability can be linked to success in any undertaking, so it's important to know what strengths and weaknesses you have.

In order to change toward healthy life habits, we need positive emotions. When you have those in place, you'll find that it gets easier for you to accomplish things—both large and small. That's because resistance no longer stands between you and the task.

Mounting scientific evidence shows how emotional health can even cure disease. Other studies reveal that negative or unstable emotions can make you more prone to catch colds because the immune system is vulnerable. High blood pressure can also be a result of emotional turmoil.

If you are seriously considering taking positive steps toward better health, and would like to join Diane, Rose, Tameka, and Tawanda on their road to wellness, take the emotional inventory along with them and follow the path that they take throughout the next seven weeks. You can find that inventory on page 175.

Before our meeting was over, I said to the women, "We know each other now. So let us all work together on this, the most important part of our journey. One of the first things I want you to do after you take the emotional inventory is to start meditating each day. Next week, I will give you some techniques to use, but for now, I want you to take thirty minutes out of your busy day to find a quiet place at home or at work, to do absolutely nothing. Find a comfortable chair and sit. Try to clear your mind and relax your body."

We were coming to the end of the meeting, and for the remaining time I answered the questions that they had. Rose, who had been taking a lot of notes, asked, "Dr. Smith, you talk a lot about speeding up our metabolism. I know at school I have heard about how some Black women have slow body metabolism and how hard it is to burn off calories. If that's true, why don't you just prescribe a diet pill or supplement to help us?" I heard Diane say, "Yeh," giving clear verbal support to what Rose had asked.

I replied by saying, "The path to wellness and weight loss should be natural. There is no quick fix for years of not taking better care of yourselves. Each of you already possesses all the tools you need to be successful without any kinds of pills.

"Most of your insurance plans don't cover them, anyway, and I wouldn't recommend these pills to you even if they were covered. Medication like this works during the time you take it, but when you stop taking it all the weight comes back on.

"Besides, these drugs can alter your moods, and that isn't conducive to making the connection between the mind and the body, which is what this program is designed to do.

"In terms of supplements, there are many that can help you lose weight. There are foods, drinks, and pills that can aid in the body's ability to burn off fat. These supplements are called thermogenics because they increase the temperature in your body, which helps you burn off fat.

Hot peppers, for example. By turning up the heat in your body, they allow you to reduce body fat. Caffeine and other foods that have ephedra in them can do the same thing. When ephedra is combined with caffeine, weight loss results. Ephedra or ma huang is a naturally occurring herb used by Chinese herbalists for some 5000 years to treat various health conditions, including hay fever and asthma.

But you need to be careful using foods and drinks with ephedra in them, especially if you have high blood pressure or heart disease. *Since ours is a drug-free wellness program, you are advised not to use any form of thermogenic supplements.* However, if you want to continue to drink coffee or tea for early morning workouts or during the day, that's fine."

As I bid them goodbye, I said, "I don't expect perfection this first week. Try to pace yourselves. Don't get down on yourself if you cheat here or there. You have seven days. I'll see you for our next session, good luck!"

## Week-One Fundamentals

1. Find a doctor and have a complete physical exam. Recruit your doctor into your wellness program. Ask if there is a woman in his or her practice whom you can partner with. If not, find a

friend who wants to achieve the same goal as you, which is to lose weight and get healthy.

2. Have your doctor work with you to write down an eight-week plan. You may use the diets and plans in Part Three of this book.

3. Start a journal and write down what you eat, and how you feel during the day. This will allow you to look at the journal later to determine what you can do better or differently.

4. Study the nutrition information in Part Three so that you can increase your knowledge about what to eat.

5. Create a solid diet plan that includes eating at least five meals a day with a total of 1500 to 2000 calories a day for the first week. Drink plenty of water, take a multivitamin, and limit the sugar in your diet.

6. Start a walking program and try to walk for thirty minutes a day.

7. Take the emotional inventory to assess what your emotional condition is.

8. Spend thirty minutes of quiet time daily to meditate. Read Part Three for techniques.

9. Prepare questions to discuss with your partner and doctor.

# *Eight*

# WEEK TWO

|         | Starting Weight | Current Weight | Total Loss |
|---------|-----------------|----------------|------------|
| **Tawanda** | 270 pounds | 264 pounds | 6 pounds |
| **Diane**   | 265 pounds | 260 pounds | 5 pounds |
| **Rose**    | 250 pounds | 245 pounds | 5 pounds |
| **Tameka**  | 231 pounds | 229 pounds | 2 pounds |

A T THE BEGINNING OF THE SECOND WEEK, the women wanted to know how much weight they had lost. I congratulated them all for making it through the first week, and for coming to the second meeting with so much enthusiasm. I weighed Tawanda first. She started at 270 pounds, and after the first week weighed 264 pounds for a loss of 6 pounds. Diane was next, and she had started weighing 265 pounds. She stepped on the scale and let out a "praise Jesus!" that made everyone smile. She had lost a total of 5 pounds. Rose, reluctant to step on the scale, closed her eyes as she stepped up onto the platform. The scale read 245 pounds, down 5 pounds from her original 250. Tameka wanted to go last. She, too, was a little reluctant, but the other women encouraged her. Tameka weighed 229 pounds, and had lost 2 pounds. She started to say, "I just can't do it." But in true community fashion, they encouraged Tameka and told her that she did just fine, and that she had another week to keep things going.

The four women had lost a total of 18 pounds in one week. This was impressive! The women had exceeded their own expectations. I noticed that at the beginning of the second meeting, while the women were standing around enjoying the refreshments, they were positive, talkative, and energetic. I could see a difference in them from their first meeting just one week ago. They were feeling optimistic about themselves. So the journey had begun: the women had not only begun to lose weight, they had also begun to feel better.

We sat down to discuss the previous week. Collectively, the women felt that most of their goals had been met. I asked them to share some of their feelings, and Tawanda was the first to speak. She told the group that the most difficult thing for her to do was to eat every four or five hours. Tawanda said, "It seemed that every time I looked up it was time to eat. It was hard for a few days because I didn't seem to get hungry too much. I kept forgetting that I was supposed to eat the first two days. But I found out if on the day before I wrote down the times that I was supposed to eat, and made my meals smaller the night before, everything went better the next day. I read labels and I think that I came close to 350 calories a meal. Sometimes I even had some food left over. For the first time in a long time, I had a goal that I could go for. In fact, I didn't really feel depressed the whole week. The goal that I have for next week is to do the exercises. I really couldn't motivate myself to do that part yet."

Diane said that she felt very hungry all week, mostly at night just before bedtime. "For some reason after I had dinner at 7 or 8 p.m., at 9 or 10 o'clock I got really hungry. I couldn't figure out why that was, until I read some of the handouts on blood sugar. One suggested that I eat a piece of fruit at night. I did that, and even kept a piece of fruit on the nightstand, but it didn't seem to be enough because I am so used to eating a sandwich or chips, or even cookies at night.

"Since I was determined not to eat a bunch of junk, for the first couple of nights I went to bed feeling totally hungry. Then I called Tawanda, who didn't think I was eating enough during the day. She and I are going to sit down and go over the calorie count to make sure I'm eating enough.

"Also, I had trouble with protein. Eating broiled chicken all the time really got boring. Do you think we can talk about alternatives to chicken? Pretty soon I'm going to start clucking!" Diane smiled and as usual, got everyone to laugh with her.

She went on, "Okay, about that exercise. Tawanda and I were supposed to meet up during the week, but we could never get our schedules going together. Either she had to work or I had something going on at the church. We decided we would have to exercise early in the morning if either of us was going to accomplish our goal. But on a more positive note, some of the church congregation want to start the same wellness program. It's funny. Get a bunch of women talking about weight loss and being healthy, and it becomes a very lively conversation. They all want to come. Can they come, too, Dr. Smith?" Diane grinned as she said this, but I suggested that Diane and Tawanda get through the program first and then Diane have the minister call me about setting up a church program in the future.

Rose was the next to share her week's experience with the group. "Well, I'm a little disappointed because Tameka and I met and walked everyday, and we didn't lose as much as Diane and Tawanda. They didn't exercise. I know we're not competing, and this is a group thing. I guess I just don't really understand the logic. We stuck to the program, and I thought we would do better. Since I couldn't wait to use the dumbbells, Tameka and I started to do the lifting exercises. We were able to work the upper and lower body.

"I did feel very good and had more energy than I'd had in a long time. Tameka and I drank water until it was coming out of our ears. We joked about how many times we had to go to the bathroom during the day. I lost a lot of water. I think that all the pounds we lost this first week were water pounds."

Tameka said at first she had problems drinking so much water. "I didn't really tell Rose, but toward the end of the week I began to cut back on the water. But Rose is a great partner. She's very motivated, and it rubbed off on me. Scheduling my day was the hardest part, and she helped me get it together. I also had trouble with my meals and did not make them the day before like you suggested. I can now see how it would be easier not to have to think all day about what I eat. That was the hardest part for me. Rose and I met early in the mornings and went to the university track to do our walking. After two days, I'm proud to say, Rose had me jogging one lap, and I haven't run in at least twenty years. It felt good. I was surprised to see so many people out there walking so early in the morning."

Diane spoke up and said, "If I run, the earth will shake!"

Tameka couldn't contain her amusement with Diane, and said, "Girl, you should see all those women walkin' out there!" Then Tameka went on with her week, "About that water, I'm just not into water. I've never really been a water drinker at all. I saw Rose downtown one day, and she had her water bottle with her. I would much rather drink soda, tea, or coffee. In fact, this week I increased my coffee intake. That water was causing me to wake up in the middle of the night to go to the bathroom. I don't remember ever having to wake up to go to the bathroom in the middle of the night.

"One of the good things that happened this past week was that I became more organized. The bad thing is that I still have a long way to go. I seem to be more organized in the job, and dealing with my sick husband is easier because I have more time. Everything is already scheduled. At my job, there are cases for me to bring to trial and I have no problem doing that. But when it comes to myself, I never know what to do first. Rose was good for me because she always had her program written down. This is the area that I plan to work on next week."

Everyone had a great deal to say about her own experience during the first week. I couldn't help noticing that no one mentioned taking quiet time. When I asked, they each said that making time for doing nothing was definitely a problem. Diane shared with the group that she simply had never meditated before and that she needed help. Even though Diane was used to praying, she found it difficult to quiet her mind so that she could concentrate on herself. The other women agreed. Before moving on to the issues that were raised during our discussion of the prior week, I decided it would be a good time to do a meditation exercise.

## MEDITATION

Strictly speaking, the word *meditation* means to contemplate, to ponder and to plan. But to those who practice it regularly, meditation also means relaxation and positive affirmations.

By meditating, you slow down the incoming stimuli so that you can get in touch with your inner self. When you calm your thoughts and relax your body, you regenerate your energy sources and calm your nervous system so that you can think more clearly about your goals. I went through the following exercise with the group:

- Make a special place for yourself to meditate. It can be a room in your house or a quiet conference room during your lunch breaks. Try to meditate at a time you are not rushed, don't anticipate any interruptions, and aren't planning any household or family events. You can sit on the floor or in a comfortable chair or couch. Take the phone off the hook or put a "do not disturb" sign on your door so you will not be interrupted for at least thirty minutes. As you get more advanced in the technique of meditation, you can accomplish positive benefits in just fifteen minutes.

- The process of meditation: Sit or lie down quietly with your arms resting comfortably. Let your hands dangle with your wrists relaxed downward. Tilt your head slightly back if you are sitting. If you are lying down, get in a flat position with your neck and head supported on a pillow. Get in a good comfortable position with your arms either at your sides or resting on your stomach. If you feel comfortable having your fingers crossed, then that's okay. Make sure that your fingers, as well as the rest of your body, are relaxed and not tense or strained.

- Desensitize yourself to outside noises: The goal of desensitization is to rid the mind and body of any outside sensations. The idea is to remove incoming stimuli so you can relax. Your brain waves will slow down and you might also feel like you can go to sleep. Eastern religious masters call this state of mind "achieving closeness to God." Your body will relax slowly, and your muscles will become less tense if you focus on removing the stress. In this state, you are in touch with that inner being that can revitalize your energy, improve your discipline, and motivate yourself.

- You should talk to yourself, either silently, or softly out loud, feeding your mind and body with positive affirmations that allow you to reach your goals and feel better. Mid-day is a good time to meditate because it gets you through the remaining part of the day. It is like taking a nap at noontime when we were young children. Early in the morning, before everyone else is awake, is also a good energizing time. At this hour, meditation can help you think about your personal goals for the day, and by focusing on yourself first, you will be better able to help others.

- Find your personal focal point. As you stare at this spot, try to free your mind of all thoughts. Don't think about your family or work. Maintain your focus on the spot you choose. Keep in mind that it may seem to move as you stare at it. While focusing, concentrate on your feet and ankles. Close your eyes and visualize your feet and ankles completely relaxed. Wait a few minutes and allow this to happen naturally. Next, focus on your calves and thighs. Feel your lower body becoming more relaxed. Do the same thing as you slowly move up your body to your pelvic area. Your mind should be clearing by this point.

If you find that you are having trouble, take your time and begin back at your feet. Keeping your eyes closed, start concentrating on relaxing your stomach and chest. Feel the way your breathing naturally slows down. Breathe in through your nose and out through your mouth. Then shift your focus to your shoulders and arms. Relax your neck first, and then your shoulders, allowing the tension to leave. Since most of the stress of our everyday lives gets concentrated in the neck and shoulders, you may want to spend some extra time concentrating on relaxing this area of your body. You should be calmer from your neck to your feet by this point. Next, focus on your face and head. Allow these areas to relax. Have your scalp relax, too. Your scalp may start to tingle like the rest of your body. That's okay because that indicates you have achieved total relaxation. Some of you may even fall asleep at this point, but don't worry. That's okay, too.

As I went through the meditation exercise with Diane, Tawanda, Rose, and Tameka, I noticed that they seemed very relaxed. Diane and Rose even looked as though they were asleep.

- Become aware of how you feel. Your body and mind are now one, free from stress. With your mind in this state, think about the positive things that you love about yourself, the attributes you feel are your best qualities and that you wouldn't change. Next, think about the goal that you want to accomplish today. In your mind, see yourself actually achieving this goal. If the goal is to go walking after work, then envision walking in a park on a sunny day. Think about the goal you will accomplish today for a few more minutes. Then begin the reversal process.

- Reverse your meditative state. Keeping your eyes closed, start with your head and face and begin to awaken the sensations in these areas. Allow the feelings to come back. Now bring sensations to your neck, shoulders, arms, and the rest of your body. Reverse the direction you took when you started your meditating until you get to your feet. Once you have resensitized your whole body, open your eyes. Stand, stretch, and take a couple of deep breaths. Reach for the ceiling with your arms and then bend down, stretch, and try to touch your toes. Always drink a large glass of water after meditating.

- Write in your journal. Write down what you thought of while you were meditating. What were your feelings, and how do you feel now? Write down your goals and how you will achieve them. Are there any thoughts you could not shake or that kept recurring? If there is a thought or experience that makes you uncomfortable or feels negative, that same thought or experience can be your focus for the next meditation. Write them down.

Meditation will help quiet your emotions. It is important that you get used to writing in your journal. It gives you a chance to look objectively at what happens to you daily and consider what you can do differently to make yourself happier and healthier. You can critique your thoughts and behaviors, making changes when you think they are warranted.

After our thirty-minute meditation session, I asked everyone how they felt. Tameka said, "That's the most relaxed I've felt in a long time." All the women agreed. We took a brief break before discussing our issues of the past week.

## MOTIVATION AND PLANNING: THE ROAD TO EXERCISE

In the next phase of the session, we discussed why it's difficult to become motivated to exercise. "It's better when you begin the day before to prepare for your exercise. Some of you already have started to do your exercises in the morning. If that's better than evenings, prepare the night before. Have your exercise clothes laid out before you go to bed. This eliminates the need to look for something to wear early in the morning. Looking for something to wear can change your mind. Wear thick socks, baggy loose shorts or sweat pants, and sweatshirts. They should be placed near your bed so that all you have to do is jump into them as soon as you get up."

Even though some of the women were not accustomed to walking or running, and one of them had never been inside a gym, they were all enthusiastic about learning. I suggested that, to begin with, *walking from one corner to the next on their blocks would be a good way to start out.*

I also showed them how to walk in place if the weather was poor. I said, "Bring your knees up as high as possible, like marching, to get the full effect of increasing your heart rate. Try to march in place for at least fifteen minutes."

I also suggested that they begin stretching and strength training. Similar to cardiovascular training, this helps maintain a calorie-burning state in your body. "By building up some lean muscle, your body will burn more calories at rest," I said. Your body continues to burn off fat, sometimes for days, after exercising with dumbbells. We call such exercise "resistance training," and it is an essential part of any program designed to change your body. Some of the many benefits of resistance training include:

- A decreased risk of injury. If you are prone to pain due to arthritis, back discomfort, and other frequent aches from various musculoskeletal conditions, resistance training will help you prevent and treat these conditions by making your body stronger.
- Increased bone density. Resistance training is better than estrogen preparations for making your bones stronger. Resistance training can delay and prevent osteoporosis—a common ailment that affects millions of middle-aged, obese women—in which bones lose density and become brittle.
- Improved work capacity. The more you do, the more you are

capable of doing. During the next few weeks of resistance training, you may feel a little sore. This is common, and your body will soon get stronger, and the soreness will dissipate. Your capacity to do more exercises and use heavier weights will increase. All you have to do is stick with the training, and the positive results will thrill you.

- Increased metabolic rate. By increasing your body's metabolism, you burn off more fat. You can eat more and not gain fat because the food is used up for energy.
- A beneficial effect on depression. As you do more resistance training, your mood will become more elevated. None of us are strangers to the stress and depression that can occur when we feel overworked or stressed. Those of you who have stress in your lives will be better able to cope with it. Resistance training and meditation can combat depression, sadness, and negative thinking.
- Improved posture. Complaints of lower back, knee pain, and other musculoskeletal alignment problems can improve with resistance training. Aches and pains have a lot to do with your posture and your bone alignment. This is why chiropractors stay so busy. Having a large, weak stomach worsens back pain. Strengthening your stomach muscles so that your posture is more erect places less tension on your back muscles so that you have less back pain. Therefore, resistance training improves posture and can help you with chronic pain.

After talking briefly about the importance of resistance work with weights, Rose offered to go over exercises with dumbbells.

For the next fifteen minutes, using two- and five-pound dumbbells donated by a local fitness company, Rose went through a total body workout. She then handed the dumbbells to the other women so they could experience how the weights felt in their hands.

Tawanda was pretty quiet during the demonstration, but when Rose handed her the weights, she said, "This is something I've wanted to do for a long time. I've always admired those women who worked out a lot and had tone to their bodies. This is just what I need." Tameka even said that she would love to see her husband pick up a dumbbell, too, even though she was skeptical that he would ever be able to really do it. Tawanda smiled as Diane handed her the weights and she copied Rose's movements. "This feels pretty good. Maybe one day I'll be able to join a gym."

## CALORIE-COUNTING ISSUES

After the brief demonstration, I went on to review some of the important information from the first meeting. "If some of you are feeling too full or too hungry during the day, chances are you need to readjust your calorie intake. If you feel too full, adjust the total number of calories slightly downward and make your meals just a little smaller. Don't skip any meals to compensate for this fullness because you will slow down your metabolism if you do so. Feeling fatigued or hungry during the first and second weeks is pretty common.

You also may need to eat more calories or eat more frequently, with less time passing after each meal. You should be eating every three hours or so. Something that might help you keep track of time is a small digital timer that you can put in your pocket or snap to your purse. Set the alarm to go off every three hours. This will help remind you that it's time to eat. Also, keep track of your calories so you can pinpoint why you might be feeling the way you do."

### Maintaining a Positive Attitude

"Because our daily lives tend to get in the way, we are sometimes confronted with situations that are not under our control. Recognize such situations, and don't blame yourself for them. Also, remember, getting healthier is not a test or contest to see who can lose weight the fastest. Although you work with a partner, it's best that you work your own program of wellness. Don't compare yourself with others. This can create negative feelings and attitudes that impede your success."

### Water

"Be sure to drink enough water throughout the day. Since your body is made up mostly of water, it makes sense to drink as much of it as possible. Water can help your body stay healthy, and it can also help you lose weight by acting as a diuretic. Caffeine from coffee and sodas can have an adverse effect on your body. Sodas can add extra calories from drinking them and cause you to lose larger than normal amounts of water from your body. With this water loss, you also lose important minerals, especially if you drink these caffeinated fluids late at night. If you are getting up at night to urinate, you may want to avoid caffeinated products and stop your intake of water earlier in the evening."

### Get Enough Protein

"In the case of protein alternatives, your goal is to have about 100 grams of protein a day. If you can get a little more, that's even better. A serving of chicken breast or lean steak will have about 35 to 40 grams of protein." I then handed the four women the following list of high-protein foods:

- Egg whites: Two egg whites have 8 grams of protein. You can actually eat a great many egg whites. Scramble four to six egg whites with salsa and fat-free cheese to make an omelet. You can also use an egg substitute found in the dairy section of your supermarket if you wish.
- Nonfat dry milk powder: A quarter cup has 6 grams of protein. This is good for making your protein shakes. Make a shake with nonfat dry milk powder, ice, and fruit for additional protein. You can also bake with dry milk powder and add it to your mashed potatoes.
- Nonfat cheese: One slice has 7 grams of protein in it. Use it like regular cheese to add protein to your diet.
- Bran buds cereal: One cup has 12 grams of protein.
- Bagels: One bagel has 9 grams of protein and only 1 gram of fat. It's better than bread for breakfast.
- One-percent cottage cheese: One-half cup has 28 grams of protein. Sliced cooked potatoes with cottage cheese is a good snack.
- Skim milk yogurt: One cup has 13 grams of protein. Substitute skim milk yogurt for butter or oil in baking recipes.
- Tofu: Depending on the type of tofu product, you can get up

to 15 to 20 grams per serving. There are tofu fat-free hot dogs that you can have for a barbecue. Add tofu burgers, pepperoni, or bacon to your next meal. I think you'll be pleasantly surprised. Tofu soaks up the flavor of the other foods, making it a pleasant addition to your meals.

- Beans: One-half cup of beans can provide 10 grams of protein to your diet.
- Protein drinks: My favorites. You can get up to 40 grams per serving. Use protein drinks like milk shakes. They can provide the nutrients and protein that you need for one meal, and they are good if you're on the run and don't have time for a complete meal.

As our meeting came to a close, I mentioned that at the following week's gathering we would go over some of the group's feelings about the emotional inventory.

## WEEK-TWO FUNDAMENTALS

- Continue to regulate and count your calories. Use recipes provided in Part Three to add variety. Use alternative sources for your protein.
- Exercise for twenty to thirty minutes. Start to plan for both cardiovascular and resistance training.
- Meditate for thirty minutes a day. Go over your emotional inventory. Keep your journal updated. Write down your feelings as well as your diet foods.
- Call your partner during the week. Try to make a time when both of you can exercise together.

# Nine

## WEEK THREE

|         | Starting Weight | Current Weight | Total Loss |
|---------|-----------------|----------------|------------|
| Tawanda | 270 pounds      | 259 pounds     | 11 pounds  |
| Diane   | 265 pounds      | 256 pounds     | 9 pounds   |
| Rose    | 250 pounds      | 240 pounds     | 10 pounds  |
| Tameka  | 231 pounds      | 225 pounds     | 6 pounds   |

AT THE START OF THE MEETING, Tawanda brought up the subject of food cravings, and it set into motion a long discussion about the types of foods everyone wanted and the different times at which they were more prone to want to eat specific things.

"I've been keeping a food journal, and writing my feelings down so that I can keep track of everything. One of the most significant things I've noticed is that when I'm overstressed or feeling down, I start thinking about eating chocolate or something very sweet, like hard candy," said Tawanda.

This is not something unusual to most people who change eating habits that they've had for many years. The urge to offset an emotionally challenged situation by eating is common among people who are stressed.

"How much candy did you eat last week?" asked Rose.

"Well, I only ate a few Hershey's Kisses, and managed to avoid the Snickers bar that I usually eat when I feel stressed. After reading about how my blood sugar dropped, I was able to understand why I wanted to eat sugar during the late evening hours."

Diane added, "It felt great to be able to talk to Tawanda about the way I was craving things and that she understood. We supported each other through our Snickers bar attacks. We finally figured out that we needed to adjust the times and amounts of food we were eating during the day, and to tell you the truth, it really helped a lot. Tawanda and I just renamed our fruit, 'Snickers,'" as she chuckled to herself.

Our look back on the past week also revealed a sense of achievement. Collectively, they all felt happier and had more energy. Tameka said that she was especially happy because she was finally feeling in charge of her life and that sticking with the program was her number-one priority. Even though she was taking time for herself, she was not neglecting the other parts of her life. She also found that by prioritizing things, she was able to deal more effectively with her disabled husband and pathological son.

Tameka said to everyone, "When I wake up early in the morning and everyone else is asleep, I feel renewed and calm. That's when I spend time with myself, thinking about what I am going to do during the day. That moment when the early morning sun peeks through the window is mine. I can actually feel myself coming back to life again. For so long I've been taking care of everyone and not myself. I've found that morning walks give me time to think, talk to myself, and work out problems."

I knew Tameka was beginning to feel good because she had begun to talk openly about her negative feelings. In the beginning, she said, she could not shake these. But during the past week, with Rose's help, she had loosened the grip of her fears that she was too old to lose weight or that she was not doing something right because she wasn't losing as fast as everyone else.

"I think one of the best things about this way of learning to take control of my health is that I'm able talk to someone while I'm going through the process," Tameka said with a sigh. "I also realized— *finally*— that if I drank more water, I felt less sluggish. What works well for me is to squeeze lemon juice into the bottle and add a couple of packets of Equal or Sweet N Low. Then the water tastes a little like lemonade. Or sometimes I like to make cold tea. I use an herbal tea bag in cold water, and it flavors the water just enough for it to taste good, without it really being a heavy tea. I just add a couple of sweetener packets to it too, and I can drink it easily."

"That's a great idea, Tameka," exclaimed Tawanda. "I would have never thought of that one."

The changes Tameka made were all worked out during the early morning hours when she had time to herself to think. Occasionally, she found time to meditate quietly in her office during lunch hour, either before or after she ate her chicken and salad. She also prayed. According to her, prayer helped her stay focused and centered on what she was doing. Tameka said, "That is my quiet time, and I'm getting to know myself again." While Tameka talked about what she did when she was alone, the others paid close attention to every word, taking mental notes for themselves.

Each of the women felt that her days were becoming exciting, and each had more energy than before. They felt more in control, and like Tameka, they approached the mornings with excitement instead of apprehension and dread as they did earlier.

"Meeting challenges each day is invigorating," announced Rose. "It's becoming fun to see if I can make it through the day without heading for the refrigerator like I used to. I even put a piece of paper on my refrigerator to mark the amount of times I open it. Call me crazy, but it's helping to keep me from eating when I'm feeling apprehensive or anxious."

Diane said, "I used to call opening the refrigerator door 'exercise' but walking is much more fun now." The room broke into laughter. Diane's humor was infectious. Each expressed that she felt that life was beginning to seem less taxing, or by Rose's interpretation, even though the stress was the same, it was becoming more manageable because each was taking time for herself and was becoming different as a result.

As for Rose, she said that for the first time in a long while, her mental alertness was returning. Even though she had always been an overachiever, Rose admitted that before she'd joined the group her grades had slipped as a result of her depressed moods. Now, she announced she had gotten an A on her biology exam just the day before, and the others congratulated her.

"It's got to be the food I'm eating, I just know it is. For the last few days, I've not gotten tired in the middle of the day and I'm able to concentrate better in classes now," said Rose with a smile. She went on to tell the group that she was diagnosed a few years before with diabetes but had not needed medicine or insulin. Since starting the new diet, Rose said that all of her finger sticks resulted in normal blood sugar levels.

Tameka, who had been in a longtime marriage, had been feeling that her relationship was in a rut. Now, because she wasn't concentrating so much on the negative aspects of her life, that too was getting better. Her son, who was lazy, started to walk with Tameka in the mornings. She stopped saying negative things to him, and as a result, he was showing her more and more respect, too. "You want to know what the best part of it all is? *I'm the one who cooks, and they have to eat what I make, so everyone is eating healthy now.* Sometimes they don't even know it. The only difference is that I make my meals smaller, and pack them up the day before, except for dinner. What they don't eat, I put in Tupperware for other meals."

Rose and Tameka, who had started walking alone, had begun to walk together in the mornings and were up to almost a mile on the track. Tawanda and Diane had increased their walking time by fifteen minutes and were now were up to forty-five minutes each time they walked. Rose talked about how they were all working together to schedule the dumbbell exercises. She wrote down a workout routine for all of them, working certain body parts on certain days. She scheduled their dumbbell work for three days during the week. Mondays were reserved for back and biceps; Wednesdays for legs and shoulders; Fridays for chest and triceps.

Fitness was beginning to feel comfortable to each of the four women. They were accomplishing things that, prior to starting the program, seemed difficult for them. They each had support from one another, which was a key element. Changing yourself is not the easiest thing to accomplish, especially alone. If you have no partner, then your doctor is your best ally.

After a short break, it was time to discuss what it meant to be emotionally healthy. "Emotional health is more important than just losing weight," I started, "because it impacts the other areas of our lives so greatly." I went on to explain that knowing when our emotions affect the way we think is something we can learn over time. "Most people who overeat, or have trouble coping with the daily stressors in their lives, also have what is called low impulse control. For example, instead of expressing anger in a healthy way, they keep it bottled up inside. Some people are not even aware that what they are feeling is anger."

"Oh, I know when I'm mad, all right! And the whole neighborhood knows it too!" said Tameka.

"Trust a lawyer to get her point across," Rose said with a smile.

Grinning from the exchange between the two women, I asked Tameka what she did after she vented her anger.

"Well doc, come to think of it, I always start cleaning or cooking. Those are the two ways I mostly deal with the stress of anger."

"That's more common that you might think, Tameka," I explained. "Anger leads to resentment and is a negative emotion that can sabotage your successes. How you handle the actual stress of the anger, and cope with the situation that made you angry in the first place, that affects the rest of your day, or even the next couple of days."

"I've never been an angry person," Diane said. "So it really doesn't affect me the way that it might someone else."

"You're right, Diane," I said, "but some people don't even realize that they're angry. Expressing disappointment with something you might have an issue with can actually be healthy. If you don't express outwardly something that disappoints, hurts, or angers you, then it can reduce your ability to cope. In my book *Walking Proud: Black Men Living Beyond Stereotypes*, I talk about this very issue. Pent-up resentment can do bad things to our health. It can make us resistant to exercise and lose control of healthy eating."

"I get angry a lot when things don't go the way I plan for them to," said Rose. "Sometimes I feel guilty for feeling so helpless. Then I get resentful and I take it out on other people."

After being quiet for a long time, Tawanda spoke. "I know what you mean. I'm still mad that I lost my mother. Sometimes I blame her for dying because I think that she could have done something about it. I never really told anyone else that before. I take it out on myself. The psychologist that I see is helping me realize that it's okay to feel guilty, and that I should just talk about it."

Diane retorted, "You can always talk to me. I'm the one everyone talks to. You should be proud that you have come so far, and honey, you can let go of that stuff. Your momma's watchin' over you right now. That should give you some strength, too!"

Some of the most important steps to healthy self-expression are as follows:

- Identifying the emotion. Are you angry, sad, scared, tired, anxious?
- Expressing the emotion. Do you stay quiet, yell, fidget, eat, clean, exercise?
- Understanding the appropriateness of the emotion. Does the way you feel actually match the situation? Do you overreact or underreact?
- Managing the emotion. Do you confront the issue immediately? Do you let it fester for a while? Do you simply try to forget it?

Tawanda began by saying, "Sometimes I get angry when I think about being alone. When my mom died, I was left all alone. I didn't do well on some of the questions on the emotional inventory test, so I guess there's a lot for me to work on. I'm in a relationship, but still feel alone sometimes. I guess when I'm angry, I don't really think of it as that. I just think I'm feeling restless. In order to understand anger, I need to identify it with how it makes me feel. In therapy, I was taught how to peel away the layers of my depression so I could get to the heart of what was really bothering me. When I'm faced with an upsetting situation, I start this peeling away process right away. As time goes by, I'm getting quicker at finding out what's really bothering me.

"When my mother was here with me, she insisted I take good care of myself. Without her to steady me, I had trouble. Now, with the help of all of you, I feel like I can express myself and don't need to eat and lie around thinking."

Rose added, "Before this program I would eat when I thought about my children. I love them and feel sad when I think about them not being with me. When I think about it too long, I start to get mad. Some of my emotion is pent up anger toward my husband, but I'm also mad at myself for marrying him in the first place. I've come to terms with this now, and it's definitely getting easier and easier to shake off the anger I feel. Tameka and I have been talking about how we tend to run away from our feelings, thinking they will go away. When I try to run or hide, I start eating. It's something I've got to keep working on."

It was Tameka's turn. "Okay, let's get this out in the open. I really resent my husband and son. My husband lies around not doing much of anything, and it's like he tries to suck me up into his way of thinking. There's always an excuse for why he is so negative toward me all the time. Maybe it's because he feels bad about himself. He even says that this group isn't going to help me. The good news is my son, who's a lot like his father, has started exercising with me. Rose and I are working on making ourselves feel more positive, and not relying on others to do it for us. If my husband who has a bad back wants to stay in bed all day and complain, then that's his business. The best thing for me is to help myself first."

Diane smiled and said, "Okay girls, I'm going to tell you my take on all of this. I leave it in God's hands to get me through my days and to give me strength. I guess it's the way I've always seen things, so it's hard for me to get mad at anyone. But I can tell you about one time I can remember being mad. Come to think of it, I got mad about food." Diane scratched her head and went on with her story. "It was at this really nice restaurant that my fiancé took me to. We were being so romantic, and the waitress kept getting the order wrong. It was spoiling the moment. I let her know that she didn't really need to be a waitress if she didn't know how to get the order right. But my fiancé was so patient, and I counted my blessings. Seeing how gently and politely he talked to the waitress, I got better hold of myself."

"Diane, I don't know how you got to be so patient, but I'm hoping some of that will rub off on me!" said Tameka with a smile.

The women's insights were full of depth and commitment to the program and to each other. *They were not only meeting goals, they were forming friendships and their own community.* It is the connection that each woman received from the others that allowed them to think and talk freely. That's why a gathering like this can create miracles of healing.

The women all agreed that they were reaching their goals and losing weight because of the program's focus on emotional health. They were feeling better about the people they were becoming.

At this meeting, I suggested that if the four women ate at defined times, their concentration could be better spent on other matters. They agreed to do this, and made a pact that would assist them in their quest. This is their plan:

First meal at 7:00 a.m.: Our group agreed that they would get up at 6 a.m. and work out. Walking for thirty to sixty minutes was the first order of the day. Then the women would eat their first meal.

Second meal at 10 a.m.: This should be a light meal or snack, with protein and a limited amount of carbohydrates. (Use the protein alternatives in Part Three to give your meals variety. If these meals are loaded in carbohydrates, especially the simple types of sugars, your blood sugar will become erratic and peak for a few hours, only to bottom out three hours later. Eating complex carbohydrates will keep you from getting tired.)

Third meal at 1 p.m.: A somewhat bigger meal than at 10:00 a.m. (Make sure you are drinking your water. Carry your bottle with you so that you can keep track of the amount you drink.)

Fourth meal at 4 p.m.: Remember, fourth at 4. This meal may be a little smaller than the meal at 1 p.m. Include a protein and a carbohydrate at this meal.

Fifth meal at 7 p.m.: The largest meal of the day. This is where your calories can be higher. If a smaller meal is all you can tolerate, then perhaps eat your biggest meal as your fourth meal.

Snack time at 9:00 p.m.: Those who exercise in the late afternoon or early evening may get hungry around this time. A piece of fruit at this time will keep your blood sugar level normal. Don't eat a lot of carbohydrates this late in the evening. Carbohydrates eaten at night tend to prohibit optimal fat loss. If you eat heaviest at the 9 p.m. meal, your body will store fat more.

One of the major reasons that attempts at weight loss fail is that they *cause* people to get hungry, or feel a bit empty, after eating. To address this, include more fiber in your meals because fiber is bulkier, and fills you up faster. Fiber is also good because it reportedly lowers the rate of certain cancers. It also takes more energy to digest fiber, so the body senses fullness in the gastrointestinal tract.

## WEEK-THREE FUNDAMENTALS

1. Make a schedule. By writing down the times you are supposed to eat, you eliminate stress. Try to stick to the plan.
2. Reduce calories by 150 to 250 for the coming week. By doing this, you can trigger your body's metabolism to burn off more fat. If you take in the same amount of carbohydrates all the time, your body gets accustomed to that level and can stabilize itself into a comfortable state of not burning off the calories. By decreasing the amount of caloric intake every other week, you jump-start your metabolism.
3. Start cutting out breads and cookies. Eat nonfat desserts, yogurts, and fruits to quench your sugar cravings.
4. Work on stress that triggers you to eat. Look at your feelings, and focus on identifying, expressing, evaluating, and managing negative feelings. Identify whether or not your emotions have anything to do with your ability to reach your goals and your journey to wellness.
5. Meditate. You should have made time to meditate by now. If not, make this a priority this week.
6. Keep a journal. Continue to write down feelings both good and bad. Look at the changes you want to make and discuss them with your partner.
7. Remember that this is the week that you will love yourself more!

## Ten

# WEEK FOUR

| | Starting Weight | Current Weight | Total Loss |
|---|---|---|---|
| Tawanda | 270 pounds | 255 pounds | 15 pounds |
| Diane | 265 pounds | 250 pounds | 15 pounds |
| Rose | 250 pounds | 234 pounds | 16 pounds |
| Tameka | 231 pounds | 220 pounds | 11 pounds |

BY THE BEGINNING OF THE FOURTH WEEK, all the women had dropped at least a dress size and were beginning to see themselves more positively. They were becoming more toned and feeling more energetic. Their average weight loss was about 13 pounds, which indicated they were well on their way to better health.

I brought fat-free frozen yogurt to the fourth meeting, and we began talking about the last week. I began our discussion by saying, "At first you thought that changing would be difficult, and you all said, 'How can I eat so many meals and at the same time lose weight?' A couple of you even said that you couldn't get out of bed early or had no time to exercise. You have accomplished things that you thought you couldn't do. Pat yourselves on the back for accomplishing these goals and relish your achievements." They all smiled and did just that, as I clapped for them.

I then explained that in the next two weeks I would again be doing blood tests on each of them to look at their lipid levels. I was anxious to also see if their good cholesterol (HDLs) had increased and their bad cholesterol (LDL) had decreased as a result of their hard work. In addition, I would also examine them, paying special attention to blood pressure and heart function.

They each complained of minor soreness, but with the exception of Rose, that was getting better as the weeks progressed. With Rose, the soreness seemed to be getting worse. She had come to this week's meeting with her knee wrapped in a thick ace bandage, and she walked with a slight limp. Knowing that she had a tendency to get overly enthusiastic about projects and accomplishing goals, I asked her what was happening. She told the group that she had strained her knee while doing double workouts each day. After hearing this, I decided to use Rose's experience to make an important point.

I cautioned everyone not to get too exuberant and careless about trying to do too much too quickly. Making big changes toward healthy attitudes and bodies takes time and patience. Already, Rose had encouraged the women to use heavier weights. Most of them had purchased 10- and 15-pound dumbbells. Although Rose had lost the most weight, I thought that if I did not say something, she might further injure herself.

I went over a few points in the meeting. "Because it is important that the wellness goals be comfortably integrated into your lives and not be a factor that creates additional stress," I said, "you should look for the following signals to tell you whether or not you need to take a step back and rethink your goals:"

- Increasing tiredness. What if, instead of feeling more energized, you feel more tired and lethargic and find yourself falling asleep—or wanting to sleep—at lunchtime. If your normal sleeping pattern changes and you're waking up in the middle of the night or sleeping too much, you might be overdoing it.

Scientists have known for years that not sleeping properly makes you tired and cranky, and may be the cause of major changes in your body. Doctor Eva Van Cauter, a professor of medicine at the University of Chicago, has been doing research in the area of obesity and abnormal sleeping patterns. One of her recent studies reports that sleep deprivation may promote weight gain. It appears that glucose does not respond to insulin when you don't sleep enough and as a result you can gain weight. So remember, *overdoing it can be almost as harmful as not doing it at all.*

- Irritability. One of the first indicators that something is wrong is your mood. A poorly integrated program will negatively impact your mood and instead of feeling great after a workout, you feel dissatisfied. So if you're feeling irritable take a second look at what you're doing. It may be time for you to take a break from training.
- Loss of appetite. It's okay not to want to eat too much, but when you don't have the desire or appetite to eat at all, this may indicate that there's a problem.
- Decreased strength. You should be getting stronger with your dumbbell training. If you aren't improving, or even find yourself becoming unable to lift, or if you are unable to walk or run the distances that you were doing the week before, you may be doing too much. Take a few days off to relax and then start again. If you find yourself tired and getting extremely winded before the workout is completed, then you're doing too much. If you're not looking forward to your next workout, again you may be overtraining.
- Your joints ache and the pain does not subside after a few days. You need to take a break from your cardiovascular and resistance-training program if you are in pain. If pain is limiting your mobility, you may need to see your doctor.

I shared these signs of overtraining with Rose, Diane, Tameka, and Tawanda, and referred Rose to a radiologist for some x-rays of her knee and encouraged her to take some time off from working out so much.

"The goal of this program is to make you healthier. If you push yourself to extremes, you will not be successful. In fact, you will be more inclined to stop what you're doing because it won't be fun. This is why many programs fail. The wellness journey is yours forever and not some fad that will cease to be a part of your life once you lose the desired weight. *It is not just about weight loss but total wellness.* Moderate and gradual changes to your personality and body encourage better long-term success than major, abrupt changes. Instead of going to a gym everyday, recognize how much better you feel if you spend an hour a day sitting quietly, enjoying TV, or reading," I said to everyone.

Diane raised her hand and mentioned that she had something to share with the group. "You know, last week I felt a little out of place. All of you were talking about the emotional inventory and about showing anger and disappointment in a healthy way. I don't feel anger or resentment. I'm happy, and most of the time I feel good about the people around me. I'm losing weight just like everyone else, so I feel like the program is okay for happy women, too. I get disappointed about some things, but mostly they are things I can't change or have no control over, so I give that over to God.

Take my fiancé, for example. He can get self-absorbed some-times, but that doesn't bother me because I know that we will get through whatever he is dealing with. In the end, he always shares his thoughts with me. What I tend to feel, more than resentment, is not always being able to assert myself more with my family and the church members who always place demands on me. I also have problems setting boundaries. Since my father is the minister of a big church, he can always find something for me to do. Sometimes he doesn't take into account my own time commitments. Church members are always knocking on the door of my office, and most of the time I can't say no to them. What are some of the ways that I can improve my assertiveness and set better boundaries with people?"

"Thank you for sharing your feelings, Diane. Many women of color—in fact, *many women*—are under some form of constant stress that hurts their health. Stress can occur when you don't feel respected and your feelings are set aside or not recognized. If you feel a need to be more assertive and to set clearly defined boundaries, it may be that your social relationships don't meet your emotional needs. By setting boundaries and reducing stress, you can reach the goals that you set for optimal emotional health. Some ways to do that are:

1. Set boundaries. Think clearly about what you expect from others, and what they should expect from you. Diane, for exam-

ple, needed to think about her parents and members of her church and decide what she wants from them. She also needs to think about the situations she's in and how to react to them. The boundaries that you set may vary depending on your situation, but the important thing is to be consistent in your approach to them.

2. Educate or inform people about what bothers you. For example, if you do not want to be disturbed at lunchtime so that you can work on your personal wellness, simply let everyone know that you won't be available during that time. There is no need to explain why. If you do feel compelled to explain your reasons, tell people about what your goals are. This will allow them to respect you and your personal time more. Since Diane's father is the minister at the same church that employs her, she may want to explain to him about the time she is expected to work and the times that she designates as her own. Inform these people in a matter-of-fact way of the new boundaries that you're setting. Be direct and precise about expressing your feelings. If the boundaries that you set are violated, let that person know how you feel. In Diane's case, she may want to let her father know that if he doesn't become more empathetic to her time constraints, she may have to find another job.

If intrusion continues, distance yourself for a short time, or longer if necessary. At lunchtime, for example, you may want to find a quiet space away from the pressing needs of others. If this tactic doesn't work, be prepared to change your environment permanently.

Remember that setting boundaries can work only if you clearly define them to others and are willing to maintain them. Give warnings of what you will do if the boundaries you set are not respected. Follow through and be consistent about what you say. The first few times you are under pressure it might be difficult to follow through, but once you have worked repeatedly to set your boundaries you'll learn to do this fairly automatically.

The first few times you try to set boundaries, it may be hard for people who already know you to respect your new rules. It's like playing a game in which rules are changed midstream. In this case, we're talking about social rules that have been going on for a long time and people have grown used to the roles they play with one another. When the social rules change, the players have to adjust.

I suggested to Diane that she might want to let her parents and the people at her church know what she is doing. By making a kind of official announcement, you strengthen your own resolve and inform people about the new rules.

3. Assert yourself in a healthy way. During our discussion, Tameka brought up the issue of assertiveness. As an attorney, Tameka had to be assertive with others, but she sometimes had trouble incorporating this same goal into her own personal life. We reviewed how to be assertive so that each of the women would have the tools she needed in case she found herself unable to set a boundary.

Being assertive helps you meet your emotional and physical needs. By being physically and emotionally fit, you will find that people respect how you're able to get what you need in social relationships. Have you ever noticed how bodybuilders or muscular police officers are viewed? People look at them with respect and give them their space. But why is that? It is not the muscles or the sway of their step. Rather, it is the attitude by which they approach others, or allow others to approach them. Their posture enables them to stand up straight and look powerful.

This works the same for anyone when he or she interacts with others. *Assertiveness is a philosophy for interacting with others. It is not the same thing as being aggressive.* By telling other people how you feel, what you are and are not willing to do, and letting them know your personal boundaries, you gain respect for yourself and convey respect for the other person in the interaction. Assertiveness is a way to ask for what you want and need. It can reflect the emotional state you feel such as anger and disappointment. An assertive interaction requires you to look at another person as your equal, guaranteeing that your opinion will be respected.

## *Rules of Assertiveness*

1. Maintain eye contact when talking to others. There's no need to feel inferior, intimidated, or shy with anyone, so maintain eye contact. When you don't maintain eye contact, you inadvertently give control to the person with whom you're speaking. When you want your feelings to matter, look the person in the eye when you talk to them. Don't look away or drop your gaze because this may indicate that you don't feel confident about what you want the other person to know and hear, or that you simply don't care.

2. Make your voice more assertive. You don't have to shout or deepen your voice, nor do you have to scare people. Talking loudly surely doesn't make the person respect you more. Modulate your voice so that it sounds firm, but approachable. Make your voice decrease in tone at the end of your sentences so that you sound more authoritative.

3. Stand up straight. Try to be eye to eye with people whom you talk to. If this isn't possible, then have the person whom you're talking to sit with you while both of you talk. When you sit, sit straight with your shoulders squared, in a posture that shows others that you feel confident about what you're saying.

4. Don't allow anyone to invade your space without your permission, and don't invade other people's space. I used to have the habit of placing my hand on a person's shoulder when I talked to him or her until one female doctor told me of how inappropriate it was.

5. Your facial expression should always reflect what you are saying. Try to look serious when what you're saying is important to you. Remember that the emotion you show to others in terms of facial expression is what you get back in return.

6. Choose the correct environment in which to practice your assertiveness. Meeting in a neutral space conveys respect. To discuss a personal issue, you may want to meet in a restaurant or coffee shop. To discuss an office conflict, consider meeting in a conference room or library. When you determine the environment in which to meet, it gives you power over the out-

come. If it's your space and you feel comfortable with it, you feel more in charge.

7. Use the words *excuse me* to signify that you want attention. When you say "excuse me," it conveys to another person that you want to be heard. This begins the assertiveness process. It may also help to reinforce this with body language. An index finger pointed straight up, when trying to make your point can get the attention that you need. Black women are sometimes portrayed unfairly as finger-pointing and head-shaking to get their point across or express their disenchantment. We laugh at this descriptive behavior that shows how sisters act when they are upset, but the truth of the matter is this form of asserting yourself can be positive in getting what you want. Further, after you say "excuse me," say "I want," or "I feel," or "I don't want." Starting your assertive conversation with "You" instead of "I" tends to cast blame on the other person, and results in a defensive interaction rather than a healthy dialogue.

8. Show empathy. Let the person know that you can imagine what he or she is feeling. For example, Diane may want to tell her father that she knows it may be difficult for him to get used to the new way she's asserting herself.

During this meeting, the women were delving more deeply into the intellectual parts of their personalities. They were becoming more health literate and understood the three major nutrients: proteins, fats, and carbohydrates. The women began to recognize what these nutrients do in the body, and they were reading food labels and counting calories.

In addition, the four women were also becoming more structured with their exercise and eating plans. Some of them were increasing their training and meditation. They were using protein alternatives in the recipes that were given to them (see Part Three).

I also had them cut back on the diet sodas, so they did not drink more than one or two a day. They had grown used to the taste of diet drinks and were consuming many during the day. The same strategy of abstinence applied to diet bars with sugars in them. Though these supplements claim nutritional value, they have a great deal of sugar in them. Replace these diet supplements with fruit, and the sodas with water.

## WEEK-FOUR FUNDAMENTALS

1. Schedule a doctor's appointment for week six. You need to get a physical exam that includes blood tests. Make sure blood pressure and cholesterol levels are specifically tested. If these are not better than your first tests, have your doctor review what you're doing.

2. Look for signs of overtraining. Don't overdo it. Remember to set up time for relaxation. If you take a break from your cardiovascular and weight lifting, make sure that you maintain a strict diet. If your diet is making you stale, it's okay to cheat one day of the week. Have those cookies that you've been dying to have, but then start your diet again the next day. Stepping away from your program and relaxing and reflecting on yourself and what you have been doing can jump-start your enthusiasm.

3. Keep your emotional health in check. Practice reducing the stress in your life. Work on setting boundaries and being more assertive. Remember to respect those you interact with and empathize with them by placing yourself in their shoes. Educate the people you interact with about your needs.

4. Start cutting sugar from your diet. Look for sugar replacements like sugar-free ice pops, sugar-free desserts, and fruit to squelch your sugar cravings. If sugar is a must, try fat-free, low-sugar angel food cake. (See Part Three for additional recipes that can help you.)

5. Get adequate rest and sleep. Allow your body and your mood to tell you how well you're progressing on your journey toward wellness.

6. Keep your journal up to date. Write down your feelings about your emotional health. Look for negative coping mechanisms that may be impeding you from reaching your goals such as:
   - Alcohol or drug use
   - Social withdrawal and or hibernation

- Procrastination
- Oversleeping
- Overeating or binging

7. Exercise or meet with your partner at least two days a week. Discuss with your partner positive coping mechanisms that can replace negative ones. Some of the better positive coping mechanisms are:

- Exercising more frequently (but not overtraining)
- Incorporating relaxation into your everyday schedule
- Being aware of perceptions and how you are feeling
- Challenging your negative perceptions and replacing them with positive ones
- Talking with friends and becoming more social—laughter will combat misery!
- Eating a balanced, nutritious diet low in carbohydrates

By discussing these coping mechanisms with your partner, you will be able to reduce the stress in your life. Regular exercise is a prime stress-reliever because it burns off the adrenaline released in your body. Adrenaline is the speedlike hormone secreted when your body is in the fight-or-flight mode. It causes stress on your blood vessels as well as stress on the mind. Exercise controls levels of hormones so that you feel better.

Forms of active relaxation include massage, yoga, stretching, steam baths, saunas, or simply going to a movie alone so that you can eat fat-free popcorn and drink diet soda unmolested. Your body, spirit, and mind all need to recuperate so you can rejuvenate your total energy stores. Our wellness journey should not be something from which you burn out, but something that is everlastingly present, that will help you for the rest of your life. Be good to yourself this week.

# *Eleven*

# WEEK FIVE

|  | Starting Weight | Current Weight | Total Loss |
|---|---|---|---|
| Tawanda | 270 pounds | 251 pounds | 19 pounds |
| Diane | 265 pounds | 243 pounds | 22 pounds |
| Rose | 250 pounds | 227 pounds | 23 pounds |
| Tameka | 231 pounds | 217 pounds | 14 pounds |

THOUGH THE WOMEN HAD BEEN extremely enthusiastic for the past month, they didn't seem so at the start of this meeting. They sparked up, though, when I showed them the photos of themselves taken the first week. They all were amazed! Weight reductions are usually noticeable after a 10-pound loss. Many of the women had lost 20 pounds and more, so seeing the changes excited and energized them.

The before-and-after pictures are tools many athletes use to help them monitor their progress. The before picture can be placed on the refrigerator door to motivate you. It also lets you see how far you've come. Self-monitoring can be done daily, by writing in your journal and looking back on what you wrote to assess whether or not you reached goals or changed your feelings since your last writings. Self-monitoring has a positive affect on your ability to attain nutritional and fitness goals because it provides hard proof of progress.

## THE STAGES OF CHANGE

Once the meeting got underway, Tameka revealed why the women were a little lackluster and reticent tonight. Several felt they weren't losing as much weight as they were at the beginning of the program. I told them that it was normal and natural to feel this way midway through a fitness program. "First of all," I said, "people will lose weight quickly in the beginning. That weight is mostly excess water. You will tend to lose excess water when you start eating more protein, too. Just remember this: for every gram of protein you eat, you lose 9 grams of fluid; for every gram of carbohydrate you eat, you only lose 4 grams of fluid. So, the more carbohydrates you eat, the more water you retain, and the more protein you eat, the more fluid you will lose.

The plateau you have all hit will last only a short time so it's important to just ride it out and know that after a brief period, you will lose weight again, sometimes at a faster rate than before."

Tameka noted that the body could really be a well-oiled machine and I said, "Oh yes! Our body's biochemical makeup tends to adjust itself to its environment. For example, if it's cold outside, your body will attempt to increase its temperature. It's like when you turn up a thermostat in your cold house, and it takes time to get warm; so do our bodies. You have changed the way you relate to your environment. You eat differently and exercise.

Now biochemistry has to catch up. This is what happens during the plateau period. *Understand that change is a process and may not occur immediately.* Change is like climbing a stepladder. Each step of the ladder is like a level of change in your life. Some of us move up the ladder faster than others. Some may even pause on a ladder step, perhaps savoring the step or maybe afraid to go any farther. This pause is only a plateau until you continue your move forward or upward to your goal.

Don't worry about pausing. You will get more comfortable with that. What's important is that you don't climb back down the ladder of your goals. If you do, just know that taking that step back up should be your first priority."

Here is the process that nearly everyone goes through when they are attempting to change their lives. Climbing your own ladder of success requires going through a predictable series of steps that others before have taken to bring about lifestyle and behavioral change. You can trace these steps to the following:

1. Precontemplation. This is when you first came to the realization that you had a problem and needed to change. It's the hardest step of all because it forces you to intimately look at yourself. Early on, I had made each of the women aware of her problem. A couple of the women became defensive, but were willing to listen to what I was saying. At first they had to convince themselves that something was wrong. Recognizing poor lifestyle habits is one thing; acting to fix them is another altogether. What you have to do is be receptive. No one is perfect. Precontemplation is where everyone starts, whether the goal is to lose weight or something else.

2. Contemplation. The comfortable person inside of us doesn't want to change and wants to remain the same. In our conscious minds, we have accepted the need for change. But in our subconscious mind, we fear the unknown. We realize that there's a gap between where we are now and where we want to be. Change makes sense, but there's conflict.

   A war rages between the inner personalities, the conscious and the subconscious mind, the ideal self, the person that you want to be who is fit and healthy, and the person you presently are. Your conscious mind infuses you with negative reasons that rationalize why it's okay to remain as you are. These negative strategies reinforce resistance to change. The worst-case scenario is that you resign yourself: "I just can't change."

   Many Black women think and say: "Our men like us fat." Such negative conscious or subconscious thoughts can make us give up our own desires so that we can fit the stereotype that others want for us. So when we change, we journey into the unknown and we feel fear, but that's okay, too. Change can be frightening, yes, but only when we overcome this conflict of negativity can we be the people we want to be.

3. Preparation. This is the step you were at when you decided to
   act. You overcame your negative energy. In the case of the
   four women in this book, each signed up for the program
   and was ready to start on her journey. They defined their
   goals and made a plan for action. Each accepted that there
   may be some pain at first, but understood that there's no gain
   without pain. Showing up for the journey was their first step
   to success.

4. Action. Your positive emotional energy is transformed into
   action. You start, decide to fight forward, and resist any
   future negative strategies. Health education is a major factor
   in this step. It begins when your doctor helps create your plan
   and gives you new health information. In *Healthy People
   2000,* the federal government set a lofty goal for doctors to
   help their patients. They reported that only 24 percent of
   family doctors provided nutritional assessments and counseling education.

   Most doctors think it's a formidable obstacle to help
   patients change their living habits. But the federal government
   recommends that we help patients set goals, monitor their
   progress, and follow-up with them. By meeting your doctor
   halfway—or more than halfway—you contract to develop
   healthy habits in your lives.

5. Maintenance. In this step, you maintain forward movement on
   your journey to wellness. Maintenance is an ongoing commitment to your goal, perpetuated by motivating and loving yourself, regardless. When we look at before and after pictures, your
   psychological image of yourself changes, which makes the
   result worth the effort.

   As you begin genuinely to love your new self, you are better able to maintain a fixed action plan. At this stage, there is
   no worrying about whether or not you are plateauing or
   regressing. You know that working toward your goal is a daily
   issue, and not some event you must do at once.

## TIGHTENING THE BELLY

After talking about the stages of change, Diane asked a question that I thought was important to discuss. She said, "I have made a lot of changes, especially to my body. I have lost a lot of weight but have a problem with my stomach. It's still loose. My arms are getting smaller and more toned, but I still have this stomach. What can I do?"

To help the women understand the physical changes to their bodies, I explained that "The abdominal area is always a sensitive topic for all women. Men too find that this is often the last area that we lose weight in. In order to see results in this area, our maintenance step must balance good nutrition with cardiovascular training. When I was training for my contest, I was on the last leg of my training and had four weeks remaining until the contest. I followed sound nutritional practice, did my cardiovascular work religiously, and reduced my body fat to low levels. But when I went home after spending an hour or two in the gym and looked in the mirror, I still had this big belly. I told myself it was okay, and that's exactly what you should say to yourself, 'I'm okay.' Don't be hard on yourself.

"But I did find exercise strategies that helped me and can help you. *First, increase your cardiovascular activity.* This is important to reduce the body fat on your stomach. If you don't eat properly, and you continue to do weight lifting and crunches, your stomach will get actually get bigger, not smaller."

For those few that do everything right and still don't lose weight on their stomachs, some doctors may recommend liposuction, a surgical procedure. The American Society of Plastic and Reconstructive Surgeons (ASPRS) reports that the number of African Americans seeking plastic surgery is slowly rising. Although great results can be achieved through this technique, *I have never recommended liposuction.* Better to accept the way we are even if it means having a few extra pounds on our stomachs.

Through liposuction, the doctor removes unwanted fat from the areas you want reduced. The procedure is as follows: a hollow tube (cannula) is attached to a vacuum. The tube is inserted into small incisions in the skin. The fat is removed through the tube.

Keep in mind the procedure is not without possible problems. Death has occurred, although at a very low rate, due to blood clots and heart problems. If you are planning to have liposuction done, talk it over with family members and your doctor. It is expensive and not typically covered by your health insurance. My own recommendation is to do your best to lower fat by diet and exercise."

Making a conscious effort to eat well requires some simple strategies:

- Map out your diet beforehand, and stick to it.
- Fight those urges. Always be conscious of your willpower. Stay away from trigger foods, the ones you know will be a problem.

| Trigger Foods | Substitutes |
| --- | --- |
| Cakes and pastries | Fresh fruits |
| Cheese and cheese pizza | Pasta with marinara sauce |
| Butter or margarine | Jam or preserves, mustard or ketchup |
| Fatty fish (salmon, trout, catfish) | Shrimp, scallops, lobster, halibut, swordfish, tuna, snapper |
| Nuts | Popcorn |
| Mayonnaise | Ketchup, mustard, steak sauce |
| Nonfat yogurt and ice cream | Frozen meal-replacement shake |
| Red meat (veal, beef, pork, lamb) | Poultry breast (whole or ground) seasoned the same as red meat |
| Salad dressings with oil | Lemon or vinegar mixed with herbs, garlic, and mustard |

(For me it's glazed donuts. If I see them or smell them, I'm somewhat powerless to resist. Remember that you and only you are in control of what you eat. I ask myself, "Are you going to let that box of donuts defeat you in the battle of wills?" And I forcefully answer, "No way!")

- Keep your ideal self image in your mind when you eat. Always focus on where you want to be.
- Stop opening the refrigerator door every time you walk into the kitchen. That's what you did when you were a kid. Now, as a beautiful woman of color, walk past that door of temptation.
- Don't eat before bed. Late night eating, especially meals filled with simple carbohydrates, is taboo.
- Eat low-glycemic carbohydrates throughout the day. Slow-burning carbohydrates like beans, yams, and pasta will keep your blood sugar level constant and won't make you so hungry. High-glycemic foods like donuts make you hungry. Eating them makes you crave more.
- Eat less even when you're really hungry. Don't shop when you're hungry because you'll buy a lot of food that you don't need.
- Twenty percent concentration of fat per meal is ideal. If you add more fat to your meals, you'll have to work that much harder to get rid of it.
- Get rid of all the junk food in your house. A recovering alcoholic should not keep bottles of booze lying around the house.
- When you shop at the supermarket, avoid the bakery section.
- Tell your friends that you're on a diet, or better yet, tell them that you're on a journey to wellness.
- Compliment yourself when you do well. It's okay to compliment yourself if you don't meet your daily goals if the effort is there.
- Allow yourself a treat once a week. Eat those two donuts and get back to your program the next day.
- Don't carry around a lot of money in your pockets when you go to work. You may be tempted to buy something bad that you don't really need to eat.

- Eat soup because it's healthy and filling.
- Order salad dressing on the side. Dip your fork in the dressing first, and then in the salad. This is better because even some of the healthiest dressings have fat in them. This method reduces the amount of fat.
- Don't skip meals. You can't lose fat by not eating.
- Stay busy and get prepared for the nighttime by having a good book to read just before bedtime. Sitting around and doing nothing late at night makes you crave food.
- Get used to eating sugar-free Jell-O and other such foods. I did and you can, too. You'll be surprised how these foods can squelch your sugar cravings.

To help yourself burn off fat via cardiovascular training add variety to your workout. You can walk, dance, garden, or swim, but whatever you do it's important that you enjoy the exercise. Many activities will help you burn off fat by burning calories.

Here are some exercises and the calories expended per hour when you do them moderately:

| | |
|---|---|
| Aerobics | 400 |
| Basketball | 560 |
| Bowling | 300 |
| Golf | 350 |
| Jumping rope | 580 |
| Rowing machine | 800 |
| Running | 650 |
| Swimming | 490 |
| Tennis | 400 |
| Walking | 230 |

For more information on exercise-related topics, call the American College of Sports Medicine at 317-637-9200 (ext. 117 or 127). It's best to cross-train, which means changing from one activity to another, such as alternating cycling and walking.

For a better walking exercise, try these tips:

- Walk uphill instead of on a constant flat surface. It will be challenging, but you will burn off more fat.
- Use some of the low-impact machines. Indoor and outdoor bikes can help and add variety to your workout. The Stairmaster, ergometer, and cross-trainer machines are all helpful.
- Do shorter sessions but with higher intensity. Some of you may get tired or bored by those constant, long drawn out, training sessions. Push up the intensity by walking faster.
- Purchase good footwear. Comfortable sneakers are a must if you want to reduce the stress on your knees and back. You'll do better when your feet feel good.
- Drink plenty of water. You can't do cardiovascular training when you're dehydrated.
- Listen to your body. Don't push yourself too hard. At the first sign of being lightheaded, having nausea, chest pain, difficulty breathing, or any other unusual discomfort, stop what you're doing and see your doctor. Rest is important.

## EXERCISES THAT BURN FAT OFF THE STOMACH

Now that we have discussed the nutrition and the exercise components of burning fat on the stomach, we can look at some of the exercise issues and routines that can best do the job.

The stomach comprises two important muscle groups. The part of the stomach that we call the "washboard" part is composed of the *rectus abdominis* muscles. The love handles that we dread so much are the external and internal "obliques." Both groups, support for the stomach cavity, help stabilize the spinal column. If these muscles are weak, they can pull on the muscles of the back and cause a common ailment, chronic lower back pain.

We sometimes incorrectly define how fit or unfit a person is by whether he or she has the washboard stomach or love handles. I would caution you not to place so much emphasis on this, but if you must, the following exercises will help. But first some final tips about abdominal training:

- Exercise in the morning. The best time to exercise is in the morning, immediately after your morning cardiovascular training. Do your cardiovascular work and abdominal exercises early in the morning before you eat. Schedule fifteen or twenty minutes for the stomach exercises. By prioritizing your abdominal training, rather than throwing it in at the end of a weight training session, you'll get the best results.
- Don't overdo. Work gradually, building up to your maximum potential. Remember that overuse of these stomach muscles, just like any other part of your body, can lead to injuries.
- Don't do too much twisting at the waist. Twisting will expose the lumbar region of your lower back to spinal disc injury. What's more, doing too much bending and twisting can, in fact, make your waist wider, not thinner, by making those muscles bigger.
- When performing leg lifts, do them slowly in a controlled motion. Maintain slower descent to get at the deep fibers of your stomach.
- Work your stomach only three times a week so that you don't get bored or injured.
- Do three cycles of four exercises. You don't rest until you finish the cycle, and the rest period should be two or three minutes. Start with only two cycles and move up to the recommended three.
- Although most of the exercises can be performed effectively on the floor or on a flat bench, the use of a decline bench will increase the workload on your stomach.
- During the rest periods, stretch and tighten the muscles of your stomach and perform "stomach vacuums" to enhance control over the abdominals. Stretch your body by locking your hands and reaching as high for the sky as you can. Hold it for ten to twenty seconds, and then repeat. To get to those love handles, lean to the right while keeping your torso facing forward. Focus on keeping your waistline tight. Move slowly and don't twist.

# The Exercises
### (see part 3 for additional weight training exercises)

- **Lower abdominal cruches.** Do 10 to 15 repetitions. Lie on the floor, with your knees bent at a 45-degree angle. Bring your knees toward your chest in a slow and controlled fashion. If you're unable to do this lying on the floor, you can sit in a chair and use the same leg movements. Try to focus on contracting the lower muscles of your stomach. Return to the starting position.

  For those of you sitting in a chair or on the edge or a bench, sit with your body parallel to the chair or bench. Grasp the edges or the sides of the chair for support. Bend your knees and raise them toward your chest. Try to keep you toes pointed downward. Mentally focus on squeezing your stomach muscles throughout the movement and try not to have your feet touch the bench.

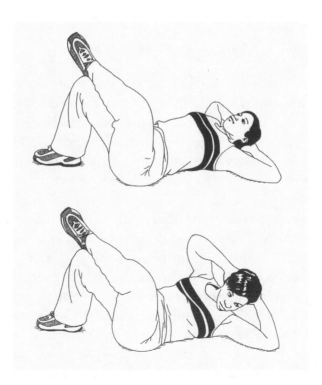

- **Leg-raises.** Do 10 to 15 repetitions. Lie on the floor or on a flat bench. For more tension and better burn on those lower abdominal muscles you can use a decline bench. If your lower back begins to bother you, sit in a comfortable chair. With your legs straight, use your hips to lift your legs until your toes are about six inches off the floor. Keep your legs straight as you lift them.

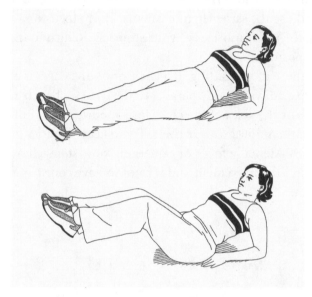

- **Side crunches.** Do 10 to 15 repetitions. Lie on the floor on your side with your knees bent and your arms holding onto either the end of a bench or something behind you. Slowly bring your knees toward your chest. Switch to the other side and repeat. Keep the movement short to reduce the tension on your hips.
- **Lying crunches.** Do 10 to 15 repetitions. Lying flat on the floor, place your legs up on a wall or a chair. Pull your shoudlers off the ground about six inches by contracting your stomach muscles. Return to the starting positions slowly and repeat. After completing the cyle once, take an active rest period. make sure you stretch. Wait two to three minutes, then repeat the exercises. It won't be too long before you're doing three to four cycles. You will get sore for a little while, but it will pass. If you're sore, you know that fat is being burned off your stom-

ach, and that's good. Perform this routine at least three times per week after your cardiovascular training.

- **Stomach Vacuums.** Stomach vacuums may in fact be the most important exercise to perform to shrink your waistline. To do them, exhale all the air from your lungs, stick your chest out, and try to suck your belly button towards your backbone. Hold for ten to twenty seconds, relax, and repeat. The best position for this exercise is to kneel on all fours. However, you can do it anywhere, even standing or driving. You can knock several inches off your waistline just by performing vacuums for a three-week period.

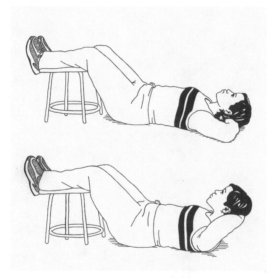

We spent the remaining session time practicing these exercises. The women caught on quickly. See you next week and make sure you love yourselves!

## WEEK-FIVE FUNDAMENTALS

1. Keep your diet strict. Try to decrease your calories by 10 percent for one week.
2. Increase your cardiovascular work to 40 to 50 minutes per day.
3. Do abdominal exercises after your cardiovascular workout three times a week.

4. Work on your emotional health. Work on change exercises, controlling impulses, and positive affirmation.
5. Meditate.
6. Keep your journal up to date.
7. Make sure you have a physical exam and blood test for lipid levels to make sure everything is going as planned.

# Twelve

# WEEK SIX

|         | Starting Weight | Current Weight | Total Loss |
|---------|-----------------|----------------|------------|
| Tawanda | 270 pounds      | 244 pounds     | 26 pounds  |
| Diane   | 265 pounds      | 238 pounds     | 27 pounds  |
| Rose    | 250 pounds      | 222 pounds     | 28 pounds  |
| Tameka  | 231 pounds      | 212 pounds     | 19 pounds  |

THE RESULTS OF THE PHYSICAL EXAMS and blood work came back prior to our week-six meeting, and they were encouraging. The four womens' bad cholesterol levels were coming down, and their overall health was improving.

During the past week, I had seen each woman individually, and even though they were still tackling some tough issues in their lives, there were more timeouts for themselves. They were ready for more information about health and nutrition, and needed to set additional goals.

Diane, who was taking medication for her blood pressure and high cholesterol, had the best results for lowered cholesterol. Her HDLs (the good cholesterol) had increased, and her LDLs (the bad cholesterol) had decreased. These changes meant that she had lowered her risk for heart disease by taking part in the program.

Besides good nutrition, exercise can help lower a person's risk for heart disease by decreasing the bad cholesterol and increasing the good cholesterol. Exercise also makes the heart stronger and lowers blood pressure. Diane was reaping the benefits.

Heart attacks are the number-one killer of Black women, and Diane was in the high-risk category for heart disease. Obesity, high cholesterol, and high blood pressure are just some of the major risks for heart disease. Diane showed concern early on about her risk for a heart attack, and I wanted to alleviate these concerns for her during the course of our program.

Statistics show that 50 percent of Black women over the age of twenty have bad cholesterol over 200, the threshold for safety. Almost 30 percent of women of color have high blood pressure. So *these women understood that losing weight, along with all its other benefits, could be a matter of life and death.* Now they wanted to learn about foods that triggered them to eat more.

## TRIGGER FOODS

Certain foods cause you to overeat. These are those tasty foods that have an unexpected amount of hidden fat and extra calories, including:

- Cakes
- Pastries
- Cheese
- Pizza
- Nuts
- Mayonnaise
- Ice cream
- Red meats
- Fatty fried fish
- Chicken

Everyone has problems with these foods.

Rose said that her body sometimes craved these foods, and she felt powerless to resist them. "My body has a mind of its own. Sometimes it screams, pizza!" Rose said animatedly.

"You're not alone," I said. "In fact, one of the reasons we eat those foods in excess is that in the past they have given us comfort from something unpleasant, or reminded us of feeling good." We often eat these foods in response to something other than hunger. We often eat them unconsciously. Potato chips may seem to just pop into your mouth. We eat these foods out of boredom, agitation, depression—sometimes even out of happiness. Generally, we do *not* eat them because of hunger."

It is important to identify those foods that are problematic for you. I admit that removing mood-food connections can be difficult. This is why I asked the women—and ask you, the reader—to keep a journal. Writing down a typical day's breakfast, lunch, dinner, and snacks can help identify problem foods and the kinds of feelings you're having when the temptation of that chocolate cake makes you act like a Zombie.

"Our goal is to replace high-fat and high-calorie foods with healthier trigger foods. *You can no longer eat without thinking first.* For example, you need to realize that when you are feeling angry or sad, you shouldn't run for the refrigerator or reach for the nearest candy bar," I explained. (See Part Three for some of my favorite trigger food substitutes.)

## High Cholesterol

We turned next to high cholesterol because that's where it all begins. High cholesterol causes heart disease because it blocks blood circulation by coating the lining of blood vessels and arteries with plaque made from fat. It becomes a hard substance that clings to the inside walls of the arteries, much like corrosion builds up inside an old pipe.

Diane was taking a type of drug called a statin to treat her high cholesterol. A greater percentage of Black women (39 percent) than white women (27 percent) have total serum cholesterol levels greater than 240 (normal levels are below 200 mg/dl). Diane's level was 280 before I put her on the drug called atorvastatin.

Clinical studies have reported that a 20-milligram dosage of this drug can lower LDLs by 46 percent. Many types of statins are on the market and you should discuss them with your doctor to see which one is best for you, if in fact, you need to take one.

In six weeks, Diane's cholesterol level dropped to 220 mg/dl, and her LDLs decreased to below 130 mg/dl (LDLs over 130 increase the risk for heart disease). Because of their effectiveness, tolerability, and safety, the statins have become the first-line agents for fighting heart disease, especially when LDLs are high. A *Journal of the American Medical Association* article, dated April 2001, shows there may be an additional protective value against fractures due to osteoporosis for women who take statins.

## HIGH BLOOD PRESSURE

Approximately fifty million Americans are hypertensive—which is to say, they have high blood pressure. The risk increases with age for women. *Hypertension is the direct cause of death in 22.8 percent of Black women compared to only 4.7 percent of white women!* This disease is linked to organ damage, resulting in heart attack, stroke, and heart and kidney failure.

At the start of our program, Diane's blood pressure was difficult to control. It averaged 162 over 100 (120 over 70 is normal). She was on amlodipine for her condition. Diane's blood pressure had improved in six weeks and was now 140 over 85, a significant improvement. Her hard work was paying off big.

The increase in her physical activity helped tremendously. Diane frowned upon taking diuretics, which I initially thought could help her blood pressure. But the limited amount of salt in her diet was a good substitute for the diuretic. A teaspoon of salt contains about 2.3 grams of sodium, and your body needs only 220 milligrams (about a tenth of a teaspoon) a day. I recommended that the women consume no more than a teaspoon of salt a day. This seemed to work in Diane's case. (See Part Three for some ways to reduce salt in your diet.)

# OBESITY

Obesity is a risk factor for heart disease. Diane and the other women were obese at the start of their journey to wellness. Their BMI (Body Mass Index) averages were well over 40. Obesity in which body fat is centrally distributed around the upper body is strongly related to an increased risk of heart disease. Over the past two to three decades, the largest increase in obesity incidence has been among Black women.

Obesity has also been associated with a decrease in physical activities, which means there is an increased risk of death associated with a lifestyle lacking in physical activity. That is one reason our wellness journey is designed to increase physical activity. As we get older, it becomes more difficult to increase physical activity, but it is certainly not impossible.

Tameka demonstrates this point quite well. She didn't allow her age and previously sedentary lifestyle to stop her from keeping up with the other women.

# DEPRESSION

Tawanda's main medical problem at the onset of the program was depression. Her physical exam and blood pressure were normal, and her cholesterol had decreased. She was feeling much better in terms of her mood disorder. Tawanda was on Prozac, a type of medication introduced in the 1990s. Compared to the older types of medications used to treat depression, Prozac has less impact on the heart and doesn't make you as tired. Prozac is also less toxic and doesn't cause that bothersome mouth dryness.

Tawanda seemed to be doing well on Prozac. In the last six weeks, her mood had become more positive and she was happier. I attributed her mood change in part to the wellness journey because she had been taking Prozac for several months prior to her enrollment in the program and had still appeared depressed. I concluded that exercise, diet, and the sisterhood connection, in combination with the medicine, were helping her a great deal.

Depression is the most common mental disorder and is twice as common in women as in men. I see many Black women in my medical practice that seem to meet the criteria for clinical depression. Some feel extreme shame just talking about how they really feel; others experience functional impairment that affects their relationships.

The most common symptoms of depression are:

- Fatigue
- Sleeplessness
- Decreased appetite
- Decreased sexual interest
- Dramatic weight loss or gain
- Constipation

These are the symptoms that bring many women of color into my office. Depressed individuals are more likely than others to develop heart disease and also to die from it. Our program was a blessing for Tawanda and can be blessing for you, too, especially if you feel stuck in your life and are generally emotionally troubled.

Studies that go back a hundred years show the link between exercise and the mood of healthy and depressed people. Most of these studies show that people who are depressed can benefit from exercise. Exercise gives people a sense of control—important for depressed people who usually feel a loss of control over their lives. Exercise also increases self-esteem and affects neurochemistry (the organ system that elevates your mood). Exercise helps discharge tension and pent-up frustrations. Tawanda needed all these benefits.

The others, without Prozac, were feeling a "high," or euphoria, that was directly related to the exercise program they were participating in. This high comes from chemicals called endorphins that are released in our brains while we exercise. These endorphins act like drugs that make us feel good, rather like the "runner's high" experienced by intensive exercisers.

## LACK OF FLEXIBILITY

Rose was completely healthy. Her knee was better, and she was back to her regular training routine. I wasn't surprised that Rose had problems with her knees because knee ailments are a common complaint for women who start exercising. According to the American Academy of Orthopedic Surgeons, more than four million Americans seek medical care for their knees each year, and many of these are women.

Women have wider hips that cause their knees to face inward at a sharper angle than mens'. This places more stress on the knees. It has also been suggested that before a woman's period, her knees actually become looser because of the laxity in the ligaments and may cause less stability for the joint. In any case, it was important for Rose to strengthen her leg muscles and do flexibility exercises to prevent any further damage to her knees.

Rose had to develop more patience about her training and about what she wanted to achieve from the program. If you have bad knees no matter what you do, running or jogging will be difficult. Low-impact exercises that don't place stress on the knee joint may be what you need. Some low-impact exercises that can help your knees are:

- Walking
- Swimming
- Bicycling
- Using simple weight machines that strengthen the quad and hamstring muscles of the thigh

Further, since many women of color are fashion conscious, in order to protect their knees, they should wear proper shoes. Avoid wearing high-heeled and pointy-toed shoes that put stress on the entire leg, including the knees. Especially if you are on your feet for long periods during the workday, a lower-heeled shoe is better. Your shoes should also have a good arch.

Purchase a good sneaker for your specific training. Cross-trainers are good if you plan to do different exercises. Pick a sneaker that is durable and that has a supportive heel and good arch.

Rose was shorter and more muscular than the other women, and she had a problem with flexibility. She would start her exercises without loosening up first. So flexibility was something that we all worked on. Tameka, too, benefited from these new flexibility exercises. Since she was over fifty years old and felt stiffness that made getting up and down a challenge, flexibility exercises were just what the doctor ordered. All women, young and old, need to be flexible. The problem is that many of us don't spend time doing flexibility exercises. Some feel that flexibility is the key to vitality. Take the following test. If you answer no to any of the questions, you need to add flexibility exercising to your wellness work.

1. Can you look over your shoulder when backing up your car?
2. Can you easily reach to a high shelf?
3. Is it easy to get down on the floor to look under a table or play with your children?
4. If you drop a pencil on the floor, can you comfortably pick it up?
5. From a standing position, can you bend down, keeping your knees straight, and almost touch your toes?

The Centers for Disease Control and Prevention and the President's Council on Physical Fitness and Sports state:

"Although flexibility may appear to be a minor component of physical fitness, the consequence of rigid joints affects all aspects of life, including walking, stooping, sitting, avoiding falls, and driving. Flexibility helps the body work better. It creates space in your joints, space for the lungs to breathe and for the organs to get their blood supply, to be oxygenated and have the toxins removed."

Following are some of the flexibility stretches we discussed and tried during this sixth week. Incorporate them into your exercise regime three to four times a week for optimum results. Set time aside so that you're not rushed, and by all means be patient; you'll get better as you continue to do them.

- **Crossover stretch for the back and the chest.** Lie on your back with knees bent, feet flat on the floor, and arms out to the sides. Cross your right leg over your left and drop both to the left. Breathe slowly and easily, letting the weight of your legs stretch your back and sides. Press your left foot down and exhale to return to center. Then reverse the same movement to the right side.

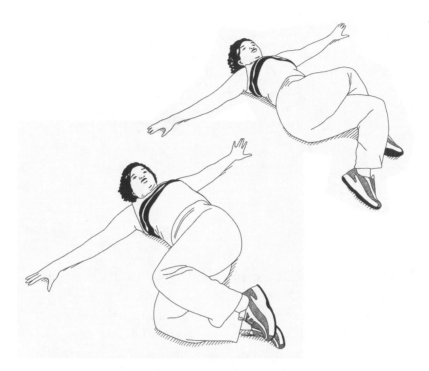

- **Arm circles for the chest and shoulders.** Lie on your back with knees bent, feet flat on the floor, hip distance apart, arms out to the sides. Drop your knees to the right. Circle the left arm down, letting the hand trail on the floor, over your legs and above your head. Repeat several times. When you hit a tight spot, stay there a while and let the muscles ease before continuing. Press your feet down and exhale to return knees to center. Then reverse to the other side.
- **Back arch for the neck and spine.** Sit backward on a chair or cross-legged on the floor. Pressing down with your hands, stretch your spine up comfortably into an arch, working your back muscles to stretch the front of the torso from neck to belly. Exhale and bring your spine back to a vertical position. Another exercise for the back and the neck is the roll down. Lace your fingers behind your head and drop it slowly, keeping the spine upright. Don't pull with your arms, but let them act as a weight to stretch the neck and upper back. Stay there, wait for the release of tension, then continue down, stopping whenever you need to.

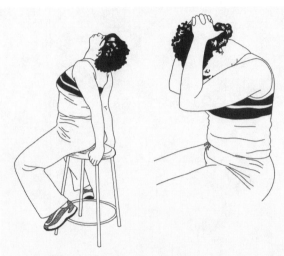

- **Hamstring stretch for the legs and hip joints.** Try to sit on the floor with your left leg bent, foot at the right thigh, right leg straight in front of you. Bend forward at the hip joint, not at the waist. If you are less flexible, don't go forward; sit up straight and let your leg muscles lengthen. That alone will stretch the hamstrings. For more of a challenge, wrap a towel around the right foot and lengthen your torso over the leg. For your quad muscles, lie on your right side with the right leg bent beneath you. Bend your left leg behind you and hold the foot with your left hand or, if you're less flexible, hold the foot using a towel wrapped around the ankle. To feel the stretch fully and completely, gently press the pelvis forward as you draw the thigh back. Then switch sides.

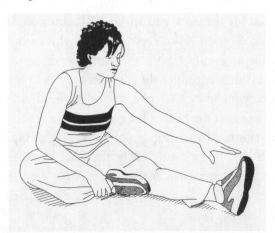

The next two stretches are for the hips, an area where the women felt tightness and discomfort while walking, running, and sitting at work for long hours at the desk.

- **Quad stretch.** Lie on your right side with the right leg bent beneath you. Bend your left leg behind you and hold the foot with your left hand or, if you're less flexible, using a towel wrapped around the ankle. To feel the stretch fully and completely, gently press the pelvis forward as you draw the thigh back. Switch sides.

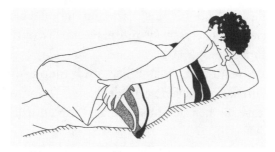

- **Hip opener.** Lie on a table, bed, or bench with your hip joint at its edge so your leg can hang down. Draw your right knee to the chest, relax your neck and shoulders, and let your left hip release. Holding the knee, exhale while drawing your left knee up. Switch sides.

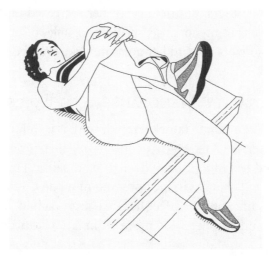

## MENOPAUSE

Tameka had a normal exam, and her blood test also showed improvement in the lipid panel. Her HDLs were higher as a result of the exercise she was doing. But Tameka had a medical condition that the others did not share, menopause.

Menopause is a medical term indicating the absence of menstrual bleeding for one year. The average age for menopause is fifty-one years. Women have symptoms of menopause between the ages of forty-five and fifty-five years because it is around this time that the ovaries begin to produce less estrogen. Symptoms of menopause include hot flashes and night sweats and mood changes. Some women experience progressively more severe disruption to sleep and daytime functioning.

Because of insomnia, irritability, and mood disturbances, women like Tameka may even seem depressed. Tameka's responsibility for the care for her sick husband and son added to her difficulty.

Menopausal women are also at risk for heart disease because of the decline in estrogen production and elevations in total and low-density cholesterol (LDLs). Obesity, weight gain, and adverse changes in body fat distribution and composition can also occur in the menopause phenomenon. In part, this is why Tameka had her weight problem.

Tameka felt a sense of failure at first because she wasn't losing weight like the others. But because of her increased understanding of what happens in menopause, she became able to set some of her fears aside and work toward her goals just like everybody else.

## SEXUALITY, MENOPAUSE, AND EXERCISE

Another problem that Tameka faced, and was reluctant to talk about, was her sex life. Many people think that sex becomes less enjoyable and less of a priority during menopause. This is not necessarily true, but changes in the body and mind do occur at this time in a woman's life and can affect her sexuality. Vaginal dryness, lowered libido, and the need for more stimulation can occur during menopause, but doesn't have to. In fact, healthy eating patterns and exercise can lessen most of these problems. Estrogen creams can help with the vaginal dryness, and for those women who choose to take estrogen replacement medication, their sex life can actually improve.

Exercise seemed to make all the women feel more sensual because they began to have a better body image. The more fit they became, the more desire they had. Studies show that exercise and dietary improvements can help women who are menopausal. The factor most consistently related to weight gain in the menopausal age group is decreased physical activity, not hormonal shifts. Tameka was more active now and, because of this, she was a happier and healthier person.

## OSTEOPOROSIS

Another benefit that all of our women were achieving was that they were lowering their risk for osteoporosis. Osteoporosis is a metabolic bone disease characterized by low bone mass, which makes bones fragile and susceptible to fracture. Although Black women tend to have higher bone mineral density than white women throughout life, they are still at significant risk of developing osteoporosis. Some of the risk factors for osteoporosis are:

- Low calcium intake
- Lack of exercise
- The absence of a menstrual period

Approximately 300,000 African American women currently have osteoporosis. Between 80 and 95 percent of fractures in Black women over age sixty-four are due to this bone disorder. Studies show that Black women consume 50 percent less calcium than the recommended Dietary Allowance (RDA).

All four women in our program took vitamin supplements to prevent osteoporosis. Each woman took in 1000 mg/day of calcium in a variety of ways, such as drinking lowfat milk, drinking orange juice, or simply taking Tums (each tablet has about 200 mg of calcium.) Exercising regularly, especially doing weight-bearing activi-

ties such as walking, jogging, dancing, and weight lifting, also work
to prevent osteoporosis.

## MUSCLE CRAMPS

Another hindrance that caused problems for the women in our program was muscle cramps and pain that some of them had during
the early portion of the journey. Rose and Diane would often complain about calf cramps. Although ice and Tylenol relieved some of
their soreness, the relief of more serious pain needed treatment with
supplements.

There are several causes for leg cramps. One common cause is
low magnesium and potassium levels. The water lost from sweating
and increased urination due to lower intake of carbohydrates causes
vital minerals to escape from the body. It is important that these
minerals be replaced.

Potassium and magnesium are minerals that have an electrical
charge. These particles play an integral role in the body's enzyme
system. They also help the body to produce energy. Magnesium deficiency, for example, can cause:

- Muscle cramps
- Leg pain
- Psychiatric problems
- Abnormalities in calcium and potassium flux
- Cardiac arrhythmia (changes in the way the heart beats)

Studies indicate that serum magnesium levels and dietary magnesium intake are lower for Black people than for whites. Certain
medical conditions related to low levels of magnesium deficiencies
include:

- Hypertension
- Diabetes
- Hyperlipidemia
- Heart disease
- Congestive heart failure
- Low potassium

- Low calcium
- Alcoholism

All are associated with low levels of magnesium, and all are disproportionately higher for African Americans.

Magnesium is a mineral that can improve strength and endurance. For this reason, when starting an athletic program, magnesium supplements and food with magnesium are vital. Studies in which magnesium and potassium were taken together have also shown performance-enhancing effects. Foods that contain high magnesium levels include:

- Whole grains
- Brown rice
- Nuts
- Green leafy vegetables

You can also take supplements that contain magnesium. In studies with athletes, muscle recovery was improved with magnesium supplements. Women who have leg cramps have lesser complaints when eating food enriched with the mineral. I told the women to be like Popeye and eat a lot of spinach. Each leaf contains 8 mg of magnesium.

Potassium, too, is vitally important for people who exercise. Cells contain potassium, which enables muscles to contract and helps nerves send messages. Potassium also helps regulate fluids throughout the body and has been shown to reduce the risk of heart disease. Low potassium levels can cause muscle fatigue. The U.S. Department of Agriculture says we need 400 mg of potassium every day. One 8-ounce glass of orange juice contains 450 mg of potassium.

Tameka, Diane, Tawanda, and Rose had two weeks to go, and tonight was more like a medical review for them.

## WEEK-SIX FUNDAMENTALS

- Maintain good eating habits.
- Introduce flexibility exercises into your regular routine.
- Continue your abdominal exercises.

- Work on your emotional health.
- Meditate.
- Keep your journal up to date.
- Be prepared to tell us how the wellness program has affected your life.
- Be sure to eat spinach and other green leafy vegetables.

# *Thirteen*

# WEEK SEVEN

| | Starting Weight | Current Weight | Total Loss |
|---|---|---|---|
| Tawanda | 270 pounds | 240 pounds | 30 pounds |
| Diane | 265 pounds | 233 pounds | 32 pounds |
| Rose | 250 pounds | 215 pounds | 35 pounds |
| Tameka | 231 pounds | 206 pounds | 25 pounds |

## Two in Their Own Words

AT THE END OF SEVEN WEEKS, Tawanda and Diane gave strong testimony to the benefits of the program, benefits I'm confident you'll experience as well.

### *Tawanda*

"I can't believe that after only seven weeks, I've lost over 30 pounds and feel like a new person. I've made great friends through this process, who gave me the support that I needed when I felt most vulnerable to failure. Dr. Smith's plan for taking care of myself really works.

"What I take away from this experience is the realization that I can do whatever I really put my mind to. Even before I met the good doctor I knew I had to change my life. At one point in my life, I felt so low that I attempted suicide, unsuccessfully. I hated my life and I can't tell you how many times I just wanted to run away from it. Too many people wanting me to do things for them, and I never had time to myself. But when I was alone I felt a need to be with people.

"I'll never forget the day that I took all of those pills so that I could just crawl into a hole and die. I felt so alone because my mother had recently died before I tried suicide. She was my best friend, and in the blink of an eye, she was gone. Sadness and resentment for being left alone filled my whole spirit. A short time later, I was also dealing with a man who was noncommittal in our relationship, and I didn't know if I loved him or not.

"Even though I had been at the same job for some time, I never really made any close relationships there. Sure, people liked me, but I had a hard time opening up to others, so they often thought I was standoffish. It had gotten so bad that one night I went to a small bar alone, and went home in a rather tipsy state. As I took off my clothes, I startled myself when I saw my reflection looking back at me in my full-length mirror. I did not recognize myself. I had let myself go. At that moment, it became clear to me that food had become my only friend.

"Most of the time when I wasn't alone, I was with my boyfriend. He was overweight, too, but constantly ridiculed me without taking a good look into the mirror himself. It wasn't helping me to feel better about myself at all. Every word he said to me was negative, and most of our time together was spent in silence. I was left in my own world of thoughts, and he eventually stopped talking to me altogether. When his friends came over, he would drink with them. I had become second fiddle in my own house.

"That's when I decided to seek help, and made an appointment with the family doctor that my health insurance company recommended. As it turned out, Dr. Smith was the one recommended, and it was like divine intervention. He sent me to a psychiatrist who helped me to deal with the loss of my mother, and the self-destructive behavior that occurred after I became very depressed.

"That is how it was. Now things are very different. I'm happy to say that I no longer associate with the man who was once my boyfriend. Happier about my life and my body, I feel healthier again. I hardly recognize the person who was afraid to look at herself in the mirror and wanted to kill herself.

"Some of this metamorphosis in my life is simply due to meeting a doctor who provided constant encouragement to me. Not only did he help me find someone to help me with what was going on inside my head, he gave me a sense of inclusion, and that was the most important thing.

"Of course, the reinvention of myself was all me. I did the work, and regained the inner strength and determination that I had lost. After I got off my butt and started working on me, my will to live and participate in life again returned. This program taught me that I was just fine the way I was, but that I had become unbalanced in my personality. Most of all, it showed me that working on me first was okay. The emotional pain and grief that I felt from the loss of my mother has been redirected into positive energy.

"I saw the signs for this program posted on a bulletin board in the doctor's office. I first thought very little about it, except that another diet was staring back at me. I always failed at them, so it didn't occur to me then that God was sending me a message and was answering my prayers. God was giving me a way to begin to change my life. There I was, scoffing at a sign that could perhaps help me to do just that.

"Sure, I knew why I turned my nose up at the idea of starting another diet. It was because I had spent a fortune on all the best-selling diet books and never thought that they spoke to me. Some I couldn't even understand, and they seemed to be tailored to everyone but Black women and our cultural needs. But despite my resistance, I made an appointment with the doctor.

"During my first office visit, I sat on the exam table and chatted with the doctor about my blood pressure and how I wasn't taking care of myself. He asked me if I wanted to join the diet program, and I let him know that he was out of his mind.

"When Dr. Smith said that I seemed depressed, I became defensive, and when he brought up the wellness program, I was angry. I had many mixed emotions during that office visit. Here was the doctor telling me it wasn't just about weight loss but about getting myself together. And here was me, who, like a lot of Black women, thought I had it all together.

"When he asked me why I didn't want to join, I told him that I

just didn't want to fail again. That's when he told me that I was joining, and that he wouldn't let me fail again. He saw the reluctance and
fear in my eyes as I nodded my head to affirm that I would try, and
he reassured me: 'The program is one where you can eat more to
lose weight, and there will be other women like you who have had
limited, or no success, trying to lose weight.'

"He called his wellness program, 'Sisterhood Connections.' I
wasn't sure how a wellness program could incorporate emotional
and intellectual health, and it sounded like hard work. And I was
nervous about working with a group. I'd always tried to work out
my problems by myself.

"The first week was the biggest challenge of my life. I was determined to first lose weight and develop some positive routine in my
life. The word *diet* made me nervous, but during that first meeting,
all of us bonded, which prevailed throughout the course of the eight
weeks.

"Before I knew it, I was exercising every day and looking forward to doing it on the next day. I'll never forget the look on my
boyfriend's face the day I told him that I was starting a new diet. It
was a cross between a smirk and a frown. Needless to say, I ignored
him, and later kicked him to the curb for his entire attitude toward
me. Working closely with other women let me see just how
unhealthy my relationship really was.

"Anyway, my first task after I dressed for exercise each day was to
call my partner Diane. Diane always told me to start my day off with
a prayer. After asking God to help me, I began with walking in place.
I attempted the push-ups against the wall and felt silly because I got
winded after doing only five of them. The crunches were a little easier. I would lie on my back and place my feet on a chair and try to
lift my shoulders off the floor.

"After the exercising, I went to the kitchen and prepared something to eat: orange juice, oatmeal, a piece of toast, and a lot of
water. I got into the habit of carrying a big jug of water with me for
the whole day. The doctor said that we had to eat these small meals
during the day. Because frequent meals would boost my metabolism, according to the doctor, I brought a small sandwich with me to
work and had an apple and some yogurt for the 11 a.m. meal. At 1

p.m., I ate a small chicken salad, and when I returned home I ate a snack. My partner, Diane, and I had to keep it simple at first, so we ate mostly the same things.

"By the time I'd been working on the program for only a few days, my boyfriend knew I was serious. After the first week, he stopped asking me with that smirk of his if I was going to get up and exercise. By the end of the first week, I knew that I had lost weight. This gave me an incentive to keep going.

"Going into the second week, I was getting better with the exercises. I'd increased the number of push-ups and crunches I was able to do and increased the time spent doing them. Exercising for thirty minutes and eating at 6:30 a.m. seemed to work well for me. The other women were all on the same routine and that made our sisterhood connection work well. In fact, the doctor didn't want us to use the term *diet program* at all. Our program was a wellness journey. I was feeling better already, and even forgot to take my Prozac for a while. We didn't want to let each other down. No one wanted to be the weakest link. I was also reading the material that the doctor gave us and was surprised at how much I didn't know about nutrition.

"By the end of the second week, I had to take my belt in one notch. I seemed to have more energy. The only downside was the soreness I felt—especially around my shoulders and hip joints. But as time went by the pain went away. As I became more mobile, my mood was better, and my boyfriend noticed the change in me. He seemed to be giving me more respect and wanted to spend more time with me and also started to ask me specific questions about what I was doing. He asked if the doctor was giving me diet pills. I wasn't ready yet to tell him that he was too late with his interest in me.

"My partner, always happy and positive, was the main reason I stuck with the program. By the third week, I had lost over 10 pounds. I went out to my favorite restaurant where people knew me. They told me I looked great and asked what I was doing differently. The process was working, and I was changing my way of thinking about myself.

"Sure, I cheated a little. I ate a piece of cake and some ice cream at a party. But nonetheless, at the very next meal, I was back on schedule. I knew that the sugar was like a drug to me. If I ate it, my body would crave more of it.

"I had to be careful also with bread. It seems to me that the traditional diets many Black folks eat are so full of grease, starch, and fat. Doctor Smith explained that once we get fat cells, we have them for life. When we lose weight, we don't lose those cells, they just shrink. I also had to control the carbohydrates in order to lose weight. I stopped eating fried foods and breads and replaced them with fruits and vegetables.

"My life was changing for the better, and all of my relationships with others were, too. By week seven, I had lost more than 30 pounds. I feel stronger and am no longer depressed. I had help from the other women by forming this sisterhood. I have gotten smarter about the things I eat, prepare better food, and understand how the body can build muscle and burn fat. All other diets never allowed me to feel so in control of my life and emotions. This is something that I can keep for the rest of my life."

### Diane

"At first I felt out of place in this program because I'm such a happy person all the time and didn't have the same types of heavy-hearted issues that the other women had. But my nature to nurture let me become a part of their lives and that has made me a better person.

"Because I'd always felt good about myself, it wasn't until Doctor Smith gave me a complete physical exam that I knew that I had to make some changes. He placed me on medicine to lower my high blood pressure and high cholesterol. But the program also had a spiritual component, and that part took some doing, too.

"My family and I are very close, and I have worked at the church my father ministers all of my life. When I told everyone in the group that my fiancé was concerned about how my weight would affect my health, they thought that I entered the program for him. However, I let them know that it wasn't true and that I actually wanted to do it for myself. I was tired of buying larger and larger clothes.

"No one ever commented on my size, and most of the people at church carried extra weight, too. The one thing that stands out in my mind about why I really joined was that one of our brothers at church had a heart attack and passed away a month before. When they found him, he was in a kneeling position, in front of the alter praying and a bottle of nitroglycerin pills beside him.

"That's when the church started to buzz about taking care of ourselves and treating our bodies like a temple. I wanted to learn how to take better care of myself so that I could help others do the same. All my life, I have lived for helping others. In fact, I was even thinking about becoming a minister, too. My mind is alive with all sorts of plans, but let me tell how it was for me.

"Before I had my physical, I never really knew how bad I was and how high my risk was for heart disease and diabetes. I showed up at the doctor's first meeting and met other women who, like me, had chosen to become healthier in their lives. It seemed that they had problems, especially relationship ones.

"Then I began to accept that I had some, too. I knew that because I had been under my father's guidance all of my life, I never really controlled what went on in my life. Don't get me wrong, I wasn't ever unhappy about this, but I knew that there was something missing when I started to learn about all of the different facets of my personality and how they needed to be balanced in order for me to be at my best.

"As God would have it, Tawanda became my partner. She was so different from me, but it seemed that we were supposed to be together. Our personalities complemented each other. I helped her be a little happier, and she helped me become a little more serious about my health. When she was emotionally flat and didn't feel like doing anything, I would pump her up, and she did the same thing for me.

"If I can lose thirty-one pounds, then anyone can. I knew nothing about exercising and eating right. I started from scratch and now I am starting a wellness class at the church for other women who need this type of program in their lives. The journey has given me a more balanced personality and a better sense of self.

"I live down in a basement apartment that my father made for me in his house. It's nice but it keeps me around them. It's the same at work. My parents are there, too. I think that I'll be moving out and going back to school. These are the two things that I wanted to do all along but never had the courage. I know that they will be sad when I leave, but I have to live for myself and be good to myself.

"I have always been very spiritual, so the meditation part of the program wasn't too much of a problem. My challenge was the physical effort that I thought I needed to succeed. By doing what the doctor outlined for us and working with my partner, I was able to overcome this fear and challenge myself. You know, it wasn't all that bad. I was able to learn how to exercise. The first couple of weeks were the worst, but after I got the routine going and began to integrate the new and exciting information into my life, it was easy. I never got hungry and I lost weight.

"The major thing that I want to say to others out there is that I didn't know how unhealthy I was and how at risk I was for heart disease and diabetes. My health literacy was limited to what I learned in high school, which wasn't much. Something that I really didn't know was that I thought that by lifting weights women would develop muscles like men. I also thought that there would no way that I could incorporate exercise into my life because I was much too busy. And like Tawanda said, I'm keeping this for life."

## WEEK-SEVEN FUNDAMENTALS

- Continue your six small meals a day. Try to cut your carbohydrates for two of the days.
- Do alternate training: walking or running one day; weights the following day. Don't forget to do your flexibility stretches.
- Work on your emotional health exercises, and don't forget to do your meditation.
- Keep your journal up to date. Plan to train with your partner and discuss some of the feelings you've had over the week.
- Set a date to go out for dinner. It's okay to cheat a little.

# *Fourteen*

# WEEK EIGHT

|  | Starting Weight | Current Weight | Total Loss |
|---|---|---|---|
| Tawanda | 270 pounds | 235 pounds | 35 pounds |
| Diane | 265 pounds | 229 pounds | 36 pounds |
| Rose | 250 pounds | 209 pounds | 41 pounds |
| Tameka | 231 pounds | 200 pounds | 31 pounds |

## TWO MORE IN THEIR OWN WORDS

OUR LAST WEEK TOGETHER produced mixed emotions. It was bittersweet for everyone to know that it was her last meeting of the journey, yet as Diane said, "We are always sisters on the road to wellness, and we don't have to meet in a doctor's office in order to continue with our new way of life."

"That's right, girl" said Tameka, "We have each other's phone numbers, and if we get sidetracked, we'll just give each other a call. Maybe even if we *don't* get side-tracked." Diane invited Rose, Tawanda, and Tameka to her church the following Sunday, and they all agreed that it would be a great way to meet up again.

It was Rose's turn to tell her story.

### *Rose*

"Several years ago, I was diagnosed with diabetes. I don't have Type I, where you need to take insulin. Mine is called Type II, and I've been taking oral medicine to keep it under control. But after the program helped me to eat right and exercise, I was able to stop taking the medicine, and the doctor said that if I stick with my new routine I may never have to take it again. The way we are all eating is very similar to the American Diabetes Association diet, too, so it's helpful to know that I can continue without having to change anything because of my diabetes.

"I have to laugh when I think about what Diane said, about all of us having different issues. She's so happy all the time. Even though she has things come up in her life, they tend to roll off of her back a little more. I think there's bound to be problems that affect us in different ways throughout life, and Diane taught me that I shouldn't let things affect me so deeply.

"My biggest issue is that my children aren't with me. I gained weight from the stress of my divorce, and from all the ridiculous court hearings that caused emotional turmoil for me. I suppose I'll be dealing with that more in the future when I go for custody. Now, however, I have better coping skills as a result of looking at all the different parts of my personality, and it's easier now for me to control my eating through the trying times.

"When the doctor recommended that I sign up for the wellness program, I was happy to have a challenge to work for. He knew that I had trained before and, even though I was pretty down on myself at the time, he felt I could add something positive to the group, so here I am. With all the studying and working that I do, I really needed to get healthier. I was at risk for heart disease and for making my diabetes worse. By the time I'm ready to go to medical school, I'll be less than two hundred pounds for sure.

"My partner, Tameka, and I were really good for each other. Sure, we butted heads a couple of times, but all in the spirit of the process. She is an intellectual like me. At first, she had trouble keeping up with me because I started with both feet hitting the ground running. Tameka told me that she was afraid that she was too old, but I encouraged her to get motivated and assured her that we were going to be great partners. We are now training together and probably will continue to do so.

"I developed a routine the first week and purchased dumbbells that were heavier than the ones the doctor gave us. I guess that I was doing too much at first because my bad knee gave me trouble. The day we went over flexibility stretches I learned a lot. This program has given me a better attitude and patience for my training and long-range goals again.

"Looking five years ahead, I have a picture in my mind as to how I want things to be, and can't wait to get there. I think it was the goal-setting portion of the program that most impressed me. Since my tendency is to get things done yesterday, the minute I started to focus on myself, I realized that I had to take things one step at a time.

"Another change came when I started to take time out each day to meditate and reflect. One of the hardest things for me is to get moving after thinking about my children, but I know I won't have the strength to fight for them when the time comes if I'm not balanced. I know God will bring my children back to me. And when that happens, I'll be at my best for them. The emotional fitness exercises help me to monitor my stress level.

"I no longer think the way I used to. My personality had gone through a transformation that makes me a better person for myself and for my children. Prior to starting the program, I was in my own head, and didn't really think too much about other people's situations. In effect, this program helped me to help other people, which is something that I needed in my life. The social interaction was probably the most compelling part of the journey, and I realize that by being social and making friends, I am able to ignore the stress so much better.

"The other day I went into the basement and pulled out some of my old clothes, ones I wore before I got so heavy, and some of them actually fit me. I can't tell you how good that makes me feel, or how glad I am to be in a sisterhood that helps me improve my mind and body."

### *Tameka*

"I'm not sure how, but this new way of eating helped heal my stomach. Before I started the program, Tums and statins were part of my everyday routine. The doctor had me undergo several types of tests and even an upper endoscopy (where the doctor places a scope down into your stomach to view the lining to determine if you have an ulcer). The results showed that I had an old ulcer that was healing and an inflamed lining to my stomach. Medicine was suggested but not really required.

"I think my medical condition was caused by the stress in my life because when things were calm for me my stomach didn't give me too much trouble. The meeting about emotions, where we discussed resentment and how it caused the body to react physically, sometimes in a negative way, helped me understand more about how emotions can affect our physical health.

"Taking care of a sick and cantankerous husband, and a son who has done much to cause me pain, had a lot to do with my condition. My emotional immune system was being bombarded from all angles, and I couldn't get out of my chaotic home life without help.

"My job as a lawyer had ceased to bring me joy and it had become humdrum. That didn't help my weight and my mood. Some of the negative changes that were going on within me were also associated with menopause. Since I was scared of how my body might react, I refused the doctor's recommendation for estrogen therapy. It just didn't seem like the natural thing to me.

"It wasn't until Doctor Smith suggested this program to me that I begin to feel a sparkle of hope. I hesitated for a couple of weeks, but decided that it was just what I needed to feel better. It shouldn't have mattered, but at the first meeting, I felt a little out of place because I was the oldest one and couldn't understand why there weren't other women my age present. Most of the women I know need to lose weight, and it's hard to believe that they weren't here, too. But the doctor explained that it was a trial group, and that the program would continue after our first eight weeks with larger groups of women.

"This program gave me the opportunity to get my life back. Although, at work I was structured and organized, I figured out that what I needed in my personal life was more control for myself. Until now it was my family who called the shots, and I responded. Once I started working on myself, my family began to back off and gave me my space. Don't get me wrong, my husband wasn't supportive of me doing something that didn't pertain to him, but he got used to the fact that I was going to do it with or without his support. They all began to come around midway through, especially when they witnessed firsthand the improvement that I was making.

"The first couple of weeks on the program I was sore as hell. Rose worked me to death, but I did not quit. I prepared my meals the night before and got up early to start my exercises. After three weeks, it seemed automatic. I could have never lost 31 pounds on my own, particularly in just eight weeks. It wasn't just the diet and exercise that did this for me, it was the emotional health and spiritual part of the program that helped me the most. The sisterhood connection gave me strength and a sense of who I was as a woman of color. I wasn't alone, but part of a group of women with purpose and deserving of health and happiness.

"Meditating and stretching with time for only me allowed me to be a different person. After a while, it really began to impact my family. My husband became less critical, and my son started walking with me in the mornings. With a toned body and a healthier personality, I look forward to practicing this lifestyle for the rest of my life. Last week I signed up for a walk-a-thon for the fight against breast cancer. It's five miles, but I have no fear because I lasted eight weeks and feel prepared for the challenge."

## FINAL THOUGHTS

With that, the women concluded their journey with me. I felt like a proud parent bidding farewell to a child as she departed for college. My emotions were mixed with sadness and joy. And behold, what a good-looking group they were as we shared hugs.

As a doctor, I have seen all types of people take small steps to reach their goals. There is a statement that I frequently use to share my sentiments about successful life journeys, and it comes from the *Big Book* used in the Alcoholic's Anonymous program. It says, "rarely have we seen a person fail who has thoroughly followed our path. . . . Many of us exclaimed, what an order, I can't go through with it. Do not be discouraged. No one among us has been able to maintain anything like perfect adherence to these principles." Like

AA, my program doesn't require perfection—just a steady movement toward one's goals.

I don't expect you, the reader, to adhere to every specific step that our women took. But I guarantee that if you make similar adjustments in your life, you cannot fail to reap benefits. The four women lost a total of 143 pounds in eight weeks. They became healthier and emotionally happier people. Diane, Tameka, Rose, and Tawanda all became more strategic about what they ate and how they reacted to stress and challenges in their lives.

I acted as their coach and counselor for the eight weeks, and during that time I gave technical advice about how to exercise properly and gave information about nutrition plans. As a counselor, I encouraged the women to talk about the experiences of their journey and was available for emotional support. The strides that these women made during the eight weeks are still being made one year later. Each of the women has become fitness centered, and each has taken other women of color under her wing to show them how to become healthier.

This is a practical program to help people, specifically women of color. *If your doctor doesn't have a program that is culturally sensitive, bring this book to his or her attention.* True, some doctors may find the program a bit unorthodox because it uses the medical model of family medicine men and women who treat the total patient in a dynamic way.

I hope these doctors will think twice. The kind of medicine practiced today has, unfortunately, left many people of color frustrated with the healthcare system. Patients are increasingly dissatisfied, and have negative impressions of a system that is flawed by cost constraints or dehumanizing treatment. Many of us in the medical community feel a strong need to rethink how we treat patients. By expanding the medical model to use the patient's own spiritual, mental, and physical resources for health and healing, perhaps we can change the negative trend of health management.

One model I've used in this program in part is the mind–body medicine model. I believe the power of the mind can help heal the body by improving how we feel and think about ourselves and how we approach our everyday lives. In *The Power of Your Subconscious*

*Mind,* Doctor Joseph Murphy suggests that when people learn how to believe in something without reservation and to picture it in their mind, they can make that belief a reality. Each of the women during this eight-week program developed her body as well as her mind and emotions. I invite other healthcare providers to become receptive to this expanded model of medical care. Try something that can help African American women reduce their risk of mortality and morbidity.

*Let me end with congratulations and admiration to the women of color who, by embracing the physical, spiritual, emotional, intellectual, and social parts of their personalities, become, at last, balanced and healthier people.*

*Part Three*

# TOOLS FOR THE JOURNEY

# *Fifteen*

## DIAGNOSING YOUR OWN EATING DISORDERS

DISORDERED EATING AFFECTS PEOPLE in various ways. Typically, the symptoms follow a progressive course from mild to moderate to serious. These questions were designed to help you identify a problem with eating. Answer yes or no to the following questions. Each question is worth one point.

1. Do you sometimes feel that if you could only lose weight, you would then be able to achieve all of your other goals?
2. Do you diet or fast as often as weekly or monthly?
3. Are you frequently depressed because you feel fat or overweight?
4. Do you frequently overeat (or frequently control the amount you eat) when you are under pressure or when you feel unhappy?
5. Would you eat more than others if you didn't control yourself?
6. Do you feel "good" or "bad" according to how much you eat, how much you weigh, or how much exercise you get?
7. Did you at one time purge (throw up) occasionally when you wanted to, but now purge regularly?
8. Does purging make you feel in control?
9. Does weighing too much (or being "fat") make you keep to yourself and feel lonely?

10. Do you use laxatives, vomiting, diet pills, or water pills to help you lose weight or feel in control of your weight?

11. Do you spend a lot of time thinking about how much you have eaten or will be eating during the day?

12. Are you frightened at the thought of eating situations where you will have to eat a normal meal?

13. Do you eat beyond the point of fullness or to the point of physical discomfort?

14. Do you cook meals for others that you won't eat yourself?

15. When you feel full, do you also feel self-conscious, self-hatred, desperation, panic, or depression?

16. Are there certain foods that you trust not to stick to you, bloat you, or make you gain weight?

17. Do you secretly eat in such a way that your meal lasts longer, or seems larger, for example, cutting each piece in tiny sections or counting each mouthful as you eat?

18. Do you feel compelled to eat when you are home alone?

19. Do you secretly crave food all the time?

20. Do your eating and weight loss activities ever interfere with work, school, or relationships?

21. Do you use laxatives, vomiting, diet pills, or exercise whenever you eat "bad" foods?

22. When you have to eat a meal in the presence of others, do you worry about how you're going to get rid of that meal?

23. Do you find that you cannot stop thinking of food and weight, that it intrudes in your thoughts much or a lot of the time?

24. Do you feel frightened of food or eating because of how you might feel afterwards?

Questions 2–8 reflect issues related to the early stage of eating disorders; 9–15 the middle stages; and 16–24 the late stages. Count the number of yes answers.

From this questionnaire, you may be able to place yourself in one of those stages. "Yes" answers in the early stage indicate problems that many people go through. At this stage, it is difficult to tell whether or not you actually will progress into the latter stages and

## How Your Body Loses Shape If You Let It

Women

17    18    20    22.5    24    32    35

Men

18    21    23.5    24.5    26.5    31.5    37

have a true eating disorder. Yes answers in the middle and late stages indicate that a problem has already developed and that treatment is recommended.

Eating disorders like anorexia, bulimia, and binge eating were once thought to afflict mostly white, middle-class females. More and more women of color are seeking treatment for these disorders. Psychologists now say Black women have begun to suffer from such food compulsions at nearly the same rate as white women.

There is nothing to be ashamed about. If you scored poorly, make an appointment to see your family doctor.

# EMOTIONAL FITNESS INVENTORY

Think about your emotional well-being in the past month. For each statement, indicate to what degree it describes your behavior or intentions.

|  | very | somewhat | little | not at all |
|---|---|---|---|---|
| I finish what I set out to do | 3 | 2 | 1 | 0 |
| I deal with things soon after they come up | 3 | 2 | 1 | 0 |
| I find it hard to anticipate difficulties | 3 | 2 | 1 | 0 |
| I do as good a job as I can under adverse circumstances | 3 | 2 | 1 | 0 |
| I avoid challenges and new situations | 3 | 2 | 1 | 0 |
| I am cautious and shy away from new tasks | 3 | 2 | 1 | 0 |
| I work to satisfy myself more than others | 3 | 2 | 1 | 0 |
| I anticipate and plan ahead to meet new challenges | 3 | 2 | 1 | 0 |
| I find it hard to get involved in what I am doing | 3 | 2 | 1 | 0 |
| I know how to say no | 3 | 2 | 1 | 0 |
| I negotiate so that some tasks are moremanageable or convenient to me | 3 | 2 | 1 | 0 |
| I do minor tasks to avoid doing major ones later | 3 | 2 | 1 | 0 |
| When things get difficult, I get tired or lose concentration | 3 | 2 | 1 | 0 |

_____+_____+_____+_____=_____

total

Add up all of your scores, and then add them across and total them.

## Analyzing Results for Emotional Inventory

33+:    Congratulations, you are an emotionally healthy individual. Your emotional health should allow you to focus totally on the physical goals of the program.

27–32:   Although you did well on this assessment, there are some additional benefits you can achieve from participating in the wellness journey.

22–26:   Meditation, and the spiritual and emotional connection with our sisterhood, should allow you to become an emotionally healthier person.

0–21:    When I wrote this book, I had you in mind. This program will allow you to take back your life and achieve those dreams that you felt were impossible. It's all about you taking care of yourself first.

## Physical Inventory

Think about the way you've taken care of yourself in the past month. For each physical issue, indicate how often each is true for you or practiced by you.

|  | almost always | sometimes | rarely | never |
|---|---|---|---|---|
| Eat breakfast | 3 | 2 | 1 | 0 |
| Watch my weight/maintain healthy weight | 3 | 2 | 1 | 0 |
| Avoid sugar | 3 | 2 | 1 | 0 |
| Avoid fat | 3 | 2 | 1 | 0 |
| Avoid salt | 3 | 2 | 1 | 0 |
| Do vigorous aerobic exercise | 3 | 2 | 1 | 0 |
| Do stretching or yoga | 3 | 2 | 1 | 0 |
| Enjoy or appreciate my own body | 3 | 2 | 1 | 0 |

| | | | | |
|---|---|---|---|---|
| Am aware of tension in my body when it occurs | 3 | 2 | 1 | 0 |
| Brush my teeth | 3 | 2 | 1 | 0 |
| Fasten seat belts in the car | 3 | 2 | 1 | 0 |
| Have a physician who knows me well | 3 | 2 | 1 | 0 |
| Would seek help for an emotional or health problem | 3 | 2 | 1 | 0 |
| Relax and take time off for myself | 3 | 2 | 1 | 0 |
| Avoid smoking | 3 | 2 | 1 | 0 |
| Avoid excessive alcohol use | 3 | 2 | 1 | 0 |

_____+_____+_____+_____=_____
total

Add up all of your scores, and then add them across and total them.

## ANALYZING RESULTS FOR PHYSICAL INVENTORY

37+: Congratulations, you have demonstrated that you are taking care of your physical self. This program will afford you time and opportunity to fine-tune your body and eating patterns. It will also allow you to be a role model to another sister.

31–36: You have a good understanding of healthy eating and exercise. The wellness journey will enable you to concentrate on those areas of need for you. You will also have purpose as a role model for others.

22–30: Welcome to our health and wellness journey. This program helps you get back on track with what is important: you.

0–21:     I had you in mind when I wrote this book. The wellness journey will offer you lifesaving information that will enable you to achieve optimal health and happiness.

## SOCIAL INVENTORY

Think of the people closest to you, and your experience with them over the past month. To what degree is each of the following statements true of these relationships? Circle the one answer that best describes these relationships.

|  | very | somewhat | little | not at all |
|---|---|---|---|---|
| The people around me will take time for me when I need it | 3 | 2 | 1 | 0 |
| Those closest to me understand when I am upset and respond to me | 3 | 2 | 1 | 0 |
| I feel accepted and loved by my friends and family | 3 | 2 | 1 | 0 |
| The people closest to me support me to do new things and make changes in my life | 3 | 2 | 1 | 0 |
| My mate accepts me sexually | 3 | 2 | 1 | 0 |
| Those closest to me express caring and affection to me | 3 | 2 | 1 | 0 |
| I spend high-quality time with friends and family | 3 | 2 | 1 | 0 |
| I feel close and in touch with friends and family | 3 | 2 | 1 | 0 |
| I am able to give what I would like to my friends and family | 3 | 2 | 1 | 0 |
| I know that I am important to the people closest to me | 3 | 2 | 1 | 0 |

| | | | |
|---|---|---|---|
| I am honest with the people close to me and they are honest with me | 3 | 2 | 1 | 0 |
| I can ask for help from my family and friends when I need it | 3 | 2 | 1 | 0 |
| I can usually find people to hang out with | 3 | 2 | 1 | 0 |
| I know that others are there for me | 3 | 2 | 1 | 0 |

_____+_____+_____+_____=_____
                                                   total

Add up all of your scores, and then add them across and total them.

## ANALYZING RESULTS FOR SOCIAL INVENTORY

40+:     Congratulations, you obviously have developed the social aspect of your personality. Your outgoing personality should enable you to do well with our sisterhood connection.

35–39:   You are socially developed; however, this program will allow you to benefit even more from working with other women who seek the same goals as you.

27–34:   The sisterhood connection is just what the doctor ordered for you to start taking care of yourself better. You will become healthier and happier by using what this program has to offer.

0–26:    When I wrote this book, I had you in mind. The program will benefit you greatly. You're not alone, and there are women just like you out there. Join us. Remember, God loves you and so do we.

## STRESS INVENTORY

Rate each item.

1=always    2=almost always    3=sometimes    4=rarely    5=never

_____ I eat at least one balanced meal a day.

_____ I get seven to eight hours sleep at least four nights a week.

_____ I give and receive affection regularly.

_____ I have at least one relative within 50 miles on whom I can rely.

_____ I exercise to the point of perspiration at least twice a week.

_____ I smoke less than a half a pack of cigarettes a day.

_____ I drink fewer than five alcoholic drinks a week.

_____ I am the appropriate weight for my height.

_____ I have an adequate income to meet basic expenses.

_____ I get strength from my religious beliefs.

_____ I regularly attend club or social activities.

_____ I have a network of friends to confide in about personal matters.

_____ I am in good health (including eyesight, hearing, teeth).

_____ I am able to speak openly about my feelings when angry or worried.

_____ I have regular conversations with the people I live with about daily living issues.

_____ I do something for fun at least once a week.

_____ I am able to organize my time effectively.

_____ I drink fewer than three cups of coffee (tea or cola) a day.

_____ I take quiet time for myself during the day.

_____ I consider myself to be more open-minded than close-minded

Add your scores, and then subtract 20.

## ANALYZING RESULTS FOR STRESS INVENTORY

0–30:     Indicates vulnerability to stress
50–75:   Indicates a serious vulnerability to stress
75+:      Indicates an extreme vulnerability to stress

If you scored low, congratulations. You have good coping mechanisms, and you should do well in our wellness journey. If your score was high, fret not, this program was designed to help you overcome hurdles in your life and aid you in coping with stress better.

# *Sixteen*

# MEDITATION

*We meditate to find, to recover, to come back to something of our-
selves we once dimly and unknowingly had and have lost without
knowing what it was or where or when we lost it.*
—How to Meditate *by Lawrence LeShan*

## WHAT IS MEDITATION?

MEDITATION IS TAKING THE TIME to get in touch with our
true nature. It is a simple effort that becomes effortless as
we do it more and more. The effort comes in taking the
time out of our hectic lives for ourselves. The rest is easy although it
may not seem so at first.

When you first begin to meditate, your mind may resist because
you are used to a constant chatter in your head. Thoughts are often
uncontrolled. We tend to worry about our jobs, finances, relationships, our to-do lists, our kids … the list goes on and on. All this
belongs to the physical world. The practice of meditation helps us
temporarily let the physical world go so that we can begin to see
ourselves as we truly are—spiritual beings.

## WHAT ARE THE BENEFITS OF MEDITATION?

You will begin to notice some benefits right away while others will
occur gradually. You will experience not only purely physical bene-

fits but also emotional and intellectual benefits as well as spiritual enrichment.

The beauty of meditation is that you stay focused only on the experience of meditating and do not think about anything else. This concentration keeps you grounded in the moment. There is no room for worries or fears. The stresses and tensions you have been carrying around are suspended and you become relaxed and able to experience inner peace and joy.

As meditation is practiced regularly, you will find that you are able to handle everyday problems in a calmer and more relaxed manner. Your coping skills will increase, and you will find a new inner strength. Your relationships at home and work will improve, and your life will become more productive.

In summary, through meditation you will experience:

- Increased clarity of mind
- Improved emotional well-being
- Increased happiness
- Increased intelligence
- Increased creativity
- Improved memory
- Improved relationships

In addition, meditation has been used successfully in the treatment and prevention of high blood pressure, heart disease, migraine headaches, and autoimmune diseases such as diabetes and arthritis. It has proved helpful in reducing obsessive thinking, anxiety, depression, and hostility.

## MEDITATION AND STRESS

We've all heard of the "fight or flight response." It is a natural defense response that prepares our bodies for running or fighting. When we perceive danger, our bodies respond and prepare to either flee to safety or fight back. Physical changes that take place include:

- Increased blood pressure
- Increased heart rate

- Increased rate of breathing
- Increased body metabolism (or rate of burning fuel)
- Marked increase in the flow of blood to the muscles of the arms and legs

The more we activate the fight or flight response, the more likely we will develop high blood pressure or some other stress-related problem—particularly if circumstances do not allow us actually to give battle or flee. Although this response is a necessary part of our makeup, it does not always serve its original purpose of protecting us from physical danger. In our modern culture, this response if often activated when the danger is not physical but emotionally or socially based. Therefore, we don't flee and we often don't fight back, but we do get anxious, hypertensive, and feel other stress-related diseases.

Dr. Herbert Benson calls the mechanism available to us to counteract the effects of the flight or fight response the "Relaxation Response." This response, by stimulating an area of the hypothalamus, results in:

- Decreased breath rate
- Decreased heart rate
- Decreased blood pressure
- Decreased sympathetic nervous system
- Decreased body metabolism

One of the ways to invoke the Relaxation Response and calm yourself is through meditation. During meditation, our body relaxes and we are free of stress and tension. Hundreds of scientific research studies done over the last twenty-five years show the benefits of meditation in relation to stress. These benefits include:

- Reduced stress
- Lowered blood pressure
- Improved health
- Increased energy
- Reduced insomnia
- Reversal of biological aging

## THE SPIRITUAL ASPECTS OF MEDITATION

Meditation helps us live a healthier, less stressful life. The physical and psychological benefits are wonderful, and many people meditate only for those reasons. But these are only a part of what meditation can do for you. Through meditation, you obtain knowledge and wisdom about your true essence.

Our physical bodies are only a small part of who we are. We all have an unseen part that is all knowing and wise and always loving. This is the part of us that existed before we came into this life and that will continue to exist after we leave. Access to this part of ourselves (called by many different names: the higher self, I AM Presence, our soul, Christ, consciousness, and so on) is available to everyone. Meditation is one way to open that connection.

During meditation, by withdrawing from the outside world and all its distractions, we begin to quiet our mind. As our mind quiets, we allow our consciousness to expand and we get in touch with our own inner wisdom. We begin to hear that "small, still voice" inside. Taking the time to open up to our higher selves can make our lives much easier. Once connected, we can begin to receive guidance on how to better live our lives. This guidance can come in any number of ways, from intuition, inspiration, "coincidences," and more.

Meditation can transform our lives. As we meditate and expand our consciousness, we open ourselves up to love and light. We begin to see things from a more loving, spiritual view. We become more tolerant of others. We find more inner peace and joy—and that inner peace touches everyone with whom we come in contact.

## HOW TO MEDITATE

There are many styles of meditation. I have outlined here the steps for a basic mantra meditation (simply focusing on an object). The process should be gentle. Do not force anything. Allow yourself to flow naturally and effortlessly. Remember that in the beginning, it is normal for your mind to jump from one subject to the next. When this happens simply refocus your attention on the object of meditation and allow it to find its own rhythm. Don't be critical of yourself when your mind wanders; it will get easier with practice and you'll find yourself having fewer and fewer disruptive thoughts.

- Find a quiet place. In the beginning, it is easier to meditate in a relatively quiet spot. This will help you "turn off" internal stimuli as well as external distraction. When you've become more experienced with meditation, you'll find that, if needed, you can meditate almost anywhere.
- Sit in a comfortable posture with the back and neck straight. Be sure it is a position that you can hold for twenty minutes. Sitting in a chair with your feet on the floor is a good position. You can also sit cross-legged on the floor or in a traditional lotus position. Kneeling with your back straight is another option. Lying down may lead you to fall asleep, so it is best to avoid a horizontal position.
- Close your eyes. This is the best way to begin controlling your wandering mind. Eventually, if you choose, you will be able to exercise control enough to meditate while walking, standing, or performing everyday activities. Breath naturally. Sit quietly for a minute or two before beginning your mantra (see the next section).
- Focus the mind on the mantra or object of your choice. Begin repeating the mantra over and over. Let it find its own rhythm. The objective is to keep the mind focused on the object of your meditation. Do not use force or tension. Do not worry if your mind wanders. When you become aware that you are thinking other thoughts, or are aware of other imagery or feelings, gently return your attention to your mantra and begin repeating it again. Do not be concerned with how well you are doing.
- Continue this for twenty minutes. In the beginning, you may want to use a soft alarm of some kind to let you know when the time has passed. Do not use anything that is jarring. In a short time, you'll find yourself automatically becoming aware that twenty minutes has passed.
- Stop the mantra repetition and take a couple of minutes to slowly return to normal awareness. Do not open your eyes or stand up too fast. Allow your body and mind to readjust.

## THE MANTRA OR OBJECT OF YOUR MEDITATION

Meditation must have an object to focus upon. Although many people concentrate on their breath, the simple breathing in and breathing out, others use a mantra. A mantra is simply a word or phrase that you repeat over and over to yourself. This is usually done silently, but can also be used like a chant. A mantra can be a meaningless sound, a religious word or phrase, or something with personal meaning to you—but always keep it positive. Mantras have been shown to have very positive physical as well as mental and emotional benefits.

The number of mantras available is endless, but here are a few to get you started:

- OM (or AUM)—This is often said to be the source of all sound and a great creative force
- HAMSA—Like the sound that you make when breathing
- HAM, YAM, RAM, VAM, or LAM
- Love
- Peace
- Joy
- I am

The object of your meditation can also be a physical object (such as a candle or a favorite item) or a mental image. You can meditate on a problem or idea, a thought or feeling, or a piece of information. Again, many people simply use their breath as a focal point.

## TAKE TIME FOR REGULAR SESSIONS

Learning to meditate takes only a few minutes, and your body will immediately start to respond. However, regular meditation is needed to gain its full benefits. With practice, your level of relaxation will deepen. Your attention span will increase. You'll become more skilled at living in the present moment. Many of the mental and spiritual aspects of meditating will become apparent over time.

## WHEN TO MEDITATE

Start by meditating three times a week for twenty to thirty minutes at a time. Good times to meditate are usually in the morning after getting up but before breakfast, or in the late afternoon or early evening before dinner.

If possible, avoid meditating on a full stomach. Meditating too close to bedtime could be disruptive to sleep. Work your way up to meditating once a day, taking peaceful time out for yourself.

## Seventeen

# HEALTHY WAYS TO THINK AND ACT

## HEALTHY WAYS TO THINK

- **Make health, not appearance, your weight and health management goal.** Achieve a healthier weight for increased health benefits. Experience has shown that ideal weights are difficult to achieve. The primary goal of any wellness program should be to reduce weight to a level where your health risks and your risk for disease are significantly reduced.
- **Normalize eating patterns.** Try to focus on healthy eating. Eating should be an enjoyable experience. The goal is to adopt a healthy attitude toward eating in addition to lowering fat and calorie intake.
- **Do not deprive yourself.** Try not to exclude any specific foods. The concept of dieting carries a lot of negative feelings of guilt such as "can't haves" or "I can never have that." Whenever you tell yourself you can never have something, you'll become obsessed with having it. If you eliminate all of your favorite foods, you may end up bingeing and eating out of control when you come face to face with those foods. Instead, enjoy those foods once a week or month and prevent the guilt that will later lead you to that dreaded binge.
- **Avoid classifying foods as good or bad.** Labeling foods good or bad can lead to such thoughts as "I'm good when I eat some

foods, but I'm bad when I eat others." You may use this reasoning to act out behavior or to demonstrate how you feel about yourself. You might think, "When I want to be bad I'll eat chips and soda pop, when I want to be good I'll eat fruit and vegetables." Or "I feel bad, so it doesn't matter if I eat a lot of cookies because I'm really bad."

- **Focus on making a healthy lifestyle change, not following a diet.** Instead of telling yourself that you are on a diet, tell yourself you are making a healthy change in lifestyle.
- **Set short-term and realistic goals.** It is not as overwhelming to want to lose half a pound this week rather than 50 pounds by the end of this year! Setting realistic goals results in more confidence, higher self-esteem, and a better outcome.
- **Make gradual changes instead of drastic changes.** It will be easier to adjust to change if done gradually. Instead of modifying all eating habits at once, concentrate on one habit at a time. Focus on changing one habit at every meal or at least once a day. For instance, if you usually have two pats of margarine on your toast for breakfast, have one pat or skip the margarine and have jam. At lunchtime, instead of having French fries with your meal have a baked potato. Just concentrate on one change at a time; it won't seem so hard that way, and you won't feel so deprived.
- **Avoid quick fixes.** You may be able to fast or starve to lose weight, but you are losing water rather than fat. You can't learn healthy lifestyle changes by starving. You will have to eventually eat and be able to make healthy food choices to maintain your weight. It's not normal to starve yourself. It is ineffective, impossible to stick to, dangerous, and a guaranteed failure. It leads to an automatic eating disorder.
- **Do not set yourself up for guilt.** The concept of dieting carries a lot of negative feelings of guilt such as "shoulds." For instance, try not to tell yourself that you should exercise everyday. That may be too drastic, and then if you miss a day or two you may feel guilty and feel like a failure. It then may be hard for you to get back to exercising. Instead, tell yourself that you will exercise at least two or three days a week, so if you exercise more than that you will have surpassed your goal.

This positive approach will prevent negative thoughts and will set you up for success. Another example is to let your weight loss goal be either to maintain your weight or to lose up to 1/2 pound a week. (You really should not be weighing yourself, but if you must then set a realistic goal.) If you lose more than 1/2 pound, great, but if you can maintain your weight, you will have met your goal by not gaining weight. It is difficult to lose 1 to 2 pounds week after week. Sometime in the future, your weight will be steady before you will start losing again. So instead of getting frustrated that you did not lose those 2 pounds that you were to lose, you can feel relieved that you did not gain any weight. You will not be setting yourself up for failure.

- **Allow for occasional slip-ups.** Nobody is perfect. Having a lapse is not failing. Falling off your diet once or twice does not mean the effort is hopeless. If you are too strict with yourself, it may eventually lead to failure. Remember it is the combination of all foods eaten over the course of about a week that counts.
- **Think positive.** Positive self-talk and an enthusiastic approach to weight management will set you up for success.
- **Do everything in moderation.** It is much easier and healthier to live in moderation than in extremes.
- **Customize your approach.** What worked for your best friend may not work for you. And what works for you today may not work six months from now. You need to decide what you need.
- **Learn from the past.** Most people have tried to lose weight before. Part of their success was that they learned from past failures. Some diets focus on weighing, measuring, and preparing food, which sometimes can cause you to be too focused on the food and lead to overeating. You may then want to succeed with a program that offers prepackaged foods.
- **Reward yourself.** Treat yourself with a massage, or perhaps a piece of gourmet chocolate, for each week that you maintain your new weight.

## HEALTHY WAYS TO ACT

- **Dieting isn't enough; exercise is essential.** Increased physical activity is essential to any successful weight management program.
- **Eat a variety of foods.** By eating a variety of foods, you will feel more satisfied. Focus on eating the serving amount from the lower end of the range for each food group.
- **Do not miss meals.** Frequently missed meals can lead to unplanned snacking and unhealthy eating patterns. You will only be hungrier for the next meal, and this may lead to impulsive eating. Eating at scheduled times will help you avoid impulsive eating. Try to establish a routine that includes three nutritious meals with between-meal snacks. You will be in better control when your stomach is not so empty. On average, weight loss winners eat five times a day.
- **Eat what your body requires.** Make sure you are taking in what your weight and activity level requires your body to have so that you have the energy and the willpower you need. For example, if you find that you can lose weight on 1800 calories a day and yet you are trying to follow a 1200-calorie diet, why not follow the 1800-calorie diet? You may lose the weight faster on the 1200-calorie diet, but the chances of staying on the 1800-calorie diet are much greater. In the long run, you may end up losing more weight by following a higher-calorie diet since you may feel more satisfied.
- **Keep a diary.** Self-monitoring is an essential part of behavioral modification and has a high correlation with success. Research shows that people who keep a food and exercise diary are often more successful at weight management than those who don't. You can gain a more realistic view of how much, and why, you eat by keeping a food journal.
- **Do not weigh yourself.** Try not to use a scale. Instead go by how you feel and how your clothes fit. It will prevent a lot of unnecessary disappointment.
- **Make specific changes.** Perhaps you will drink a glass of nonfat or 1-percent milk instead of a milkshake with your fast-food lunch, or eat skinless chicken rather than chicken with the

skin. This is an easier approach than simply saying, "I'll eat lower-fat foods."

- **Designate one place in the house for eating. Doing this will help you cut down on snacking.**
- **Do not do anything else while eating (this includes watching television).** Make eating the only event while you are eating, and enjoy what you are eating.
- **Drink up.** Add 1/2 cup of fluids today and an additional 1/2 cup every day until you reach your goal of eight cups a day. Fill an empty 2-liter soft drink bottle with water when you wake up. Keep pouring and drinking throughout the day until the bottle is empty.
- **Drink from every water fountain you pass.** This will help you stay conscious of the need to drink plenty of water.
- **Read package labels.** This will help you become conscious of the nutritional value of the food you eat.

## Cereal Box Label

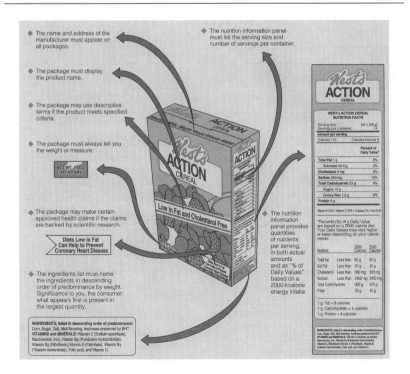

- **Become a breakfast eater.** People who eat breakfast generally feel less hungry throughout the day. When you eat a healthy breakfast, it keeps you motivated to continue to eat healthy as the day goes on. If you are not a breakfast eater, gradually build up your breakfast. If you eat only one or two foods at breakfast, add another from a different food group. For instance, if you eat fruit or drink juice, add yogurt or a slice of toast. You do not have to force-feed yourself as soon as you wake up; you may have breakfast anytime before early afternoon.
- **Start with seltzer, water, or tea.** Start your meal with a glass of water, tea, seltzer, or seltzer–juice spritzer to take the edge off your hunger.
- **Eat your meal in courses.** Begin the meal with the lowest-calorie foods such as fruits, vegetables, and salads. This will help stop those urgent hunger feelings. Finish the meal with higher-calorie foods such as bread, pasta, and meats.
- **Make meals last more than fifteen minutes.** By eating slowly, you can be more satisfied with less food. You need a certain amount of tasting, sucking, chewing, and swallowing to experience feelings of satisfaction. Eating slowly gives your body time to release the enzymes that tell your brain when you are full. It takes approximately twenty minutes for your brain to register that you have had enough to eat.
- **Put the utensil down between bites.** If you're eating finger foods like a sandwich, put the food down on the plate every so often while chewing.
- **Swallow what is in your mouth before taking the next bite.** Take time for talking, resting, or taking a drink.
- **Stop eating for a minute once or twice during a meal.** This will help break your eating rhythm and help you keep pace with slower eaters at the table.
- **If you want a second helping, wait five minutes.** The desire may go away. Also make the second helping half the size of the first. If you must have seconds, go for the complex carbohydrates—bread, rice, potato (skip the toppings), or fruit.
- **Try to leave some food on your plate.** Gradually, this will help you take smaller portions.

- **Stop eating when you leave the table.** Avoid nibbling on leftovers while you clean up.
- **Plan for a party or restaurant.** Think ahead of time what you can do to make it easier to eat right. Have a piece of fruit or a slice of toast before you go to a party or a restaurant to curb your appetite and feel more in control. Do not starve all day thinking that you will save up for the calories. It doesn't work that way because feeling hungry can sabotage even the strongest willpower. By eating just before a party, you have more control so that you can be around your favorite foods and the temptation won't be that great.
- **Plan and carry snacks.** Carry low-calorie snacks with you to avoid being hungry and prevent high-calorie temptations.
- **Do not eat from food packages.** When you nibble from food packages, you do not know how much you have eaten. You will probably eat more than you think!
- **Do not shop when you are hungry and always use a shopping list.** If you do not buy the high-calorie, high-fat foods, then chances are you won't eat them. Remember, out of sight, out of mind.
- **Respond in other ways to life's stresses.** Take a brisk walk, start a new hobby, or meditate.
- **Seek support from others.** You'll find individuals, social groups, and agencies that can help you bring about the changes you desire.

## Unhealthy Ways of Thinking

- **The perfect body and life.** Some people assume that if they lose weight, some other important goal that has thus far evaded them—a meaningful job, getting married—will suddenly be possible. Unfortunately, such goals are rarely met because of weight loss.
- **The plasticity of the body.** People assume that the body can be shaped and molded at will and that, with the purchase of the right health food or the right exercise machine, the ideal body is attainable by everyone. This, of course, is not true.

These misconceptions can have a negative effect because after failing to achieve a goal, many people experience disappointment and frustration. This yields to a negative mood, often resulting in depression. Depression may lead you into setting more stringent goals, which in turn intensifies the depression, thus starting a vicious cycle.

# Eighteen

## EIGHT-WEEK SAMPLE MEAL PLAN

I CALL THIS AN EIGHT-WEEK PLAN, but in fact I give menus only for the first four weeks. You know the drill: increase protein, adjust calories, and so on. So follow me for four weeks, then design the second four weeks according to the principles you've already learned.

### WEEK 1

#### Monday (Total—1349 Calories)

**BREAKFAST (174 Calories)**

| | |
|---|---|
| Fruit | 1 cup cantaloupe |
| Main Dish | 1/2 cup bran flakes with 1/2 cup lowfat or skim milk |

**SNACK (170 Calories)**

| | |
|---|---|
| Vegetables | 1 carrot |
| Grains | 1 small (1 oz) whole grain roll |
| Dairy/Calcium | 1/2 cup nonfat plain yogurt |

**LUNCH (395 Calories)**

| | |
|---|---|
| Fruit | 1 cup cranberry juice, artificially sweetened |
| Main Dish | 2 oz turkey breast and 1/2 oz lowfat Swiss |

                        cheese on 1/2 a small bagel with lettuce and
                        tomato
                        1/2 cup cole slaw
Dairy/Calcium           1/2 cup nonfat plain yogurt
                        1/2 cup orange juice, calcium fortified

## SNACK *(170 Calories)*
Vegetables              1 carrot
Grains                  1 small (1 oz) whole grain roll
Dairy/Calcium           1/2 cup nonfat plain yogurt

## DINNER *(440 Calories)*
Main Dish               3 oz grilled salmon
                        1 cup brown rice
Vegetables              1 cup steamed carrots
                        1 whole dill pickle
Dessert                 1/2 cup frozen yogurt, nonfat

### *Tuesday (Total—1318 Calories)*

## BREAKFAST *(166 Calories)*
Fruit                   3/4 cup honeydew
Main Dish               1/2 cup oat rings with 1/2 cup lowfat or skim
                        milk

## SNACK *(142 Calories)*
Vegetables              1 stalk celery
Grains                  1 small (1 oz) dinner roll
Dairy/Calcium           1/2 cup lowfat milk

## LUNCH *(384 Calories)*
Fruit                   1/2 cup fruit salad
Main Dish               2 oz tuna, mixed with 2 tsp lowfat mayo on 1
                        slice whole wheat bread
                        1/2 cup three-bean salad
Dairy/Calcium           1/2 cup lowfat milk
                        1 oz fat-free cheddar cheese

## SNACK *(142 Calories)*
Vegetables              1 stalk celery

| | |
|---|---|
| Grains | 1 small (1 oz) dinner roll |
| Dairy/Calcium | 1/2 cup lowfat milk |

## DINNER *(484 Calories)*

| | |
|---|---|
| Main Dish | Spaghetti and meat sauce: |
| | 2 oz cooked ground turkey |
| | 1/4 cup spaghetti sauce |
| | 3/4 cup cooked spaghetti |
| | 1/2 cup steamed broccoli |
| Vegetables | 7 florets cauliflower |
| Dessert | 1/2 cup frozen yogurt, lowfat |

## Wednesday *(Total—1370 Calories)*

### BREAKFAST *(160 Calories)*

| | |
|---|---|
| Fruit | 1 cup strawberries |
| Main Dish | 3/4 cup crispy rice cereal with 1/2 cup lowfat or skim milk |

### SNACK *(160 Calories)*

| | |
|---|---|
| Vegetables | 1/2 red pepper, sliced |
| Grains | 3 breadsticks |
| Dairy/Calcium | 1/2 cup nonfat yogurt, artificially sweetened |

### LUNCH *(405 Calories)*

| | |
|---|---|
| Fruit | 1 orange |
| Main Dish | 2 oz lean roast beef on a small whole wheat roll with tomato |
| | 6 oz minestrone soup |
| Dairy/Calcium | 1/2 cup nonfat yogurt, artificially sweetened |
| | 1/4 cup lowfat cottage cheese, calcium fortified |

### SNACK *(160 Calories)*

| | |
|---|---|
| Vegetables | 1/2 red pepper, sliced |
| Grains | 3 breadsticks |
| Dairy/Calcium | 1/2 cup nonfat yogurt, artificially sweetened |

*DINNER (458 Calories)*

| | |
|---|---|
| Main Dish | Stir-fried chicken breast with broccoli: |
| | 1/2 cup chicken breast |
| | 1/2 cup broccoli |
| | 1/2 cup carrots |
| | 1/2 cup snow peas |
| | 3/4 cup cooked brown rice |
| Vegetables | 1/2 cucumber |
| Dessert | 1/2 cup light ice cream, vanilla |

### Thursday (Total—1347 Calories)

*BREAKFAST (178 Calories)*

| | |
|---|---|
| Fruit | 2 tbsp raisins |
| Main Dish | 1/2 cup oatmeal with 1/2 cup lowfat or skim milk |

*SNACK (177 Calories)*

| | |
|---|---|
| Vegetables | 4 slices tomato |
| Grains | 1 granola bar, regular |
| Dairy/Calcium | 1 packet hot cocoa, artificially sweetened |

*LUNCH (374 Calories)*

| | |
|---|---|
| Fruit | 1/2 medium banana |
| Main Dish | 1/2 medium pita bread stuffed with 1/4 cup hummus, lettuce, and tomato |
| Dairy/Calcium | 1 packet hot cocoa, artificially sweetened |
| | 1/4 cup fat-free ricotta cheese |

*SNACK (177 Calories)*

| | |
|---|---|
| Vegetables | 4 slices tomatoes |
| Grains | 1 granola bar, regular |
| Dairy/Calcium | 1 packet hot cocoa, artificially sweetened |

*DINNER (441 Calories)*

| | |
|---|---|
| Main Dish | 1 beef pepper steak frozen entrée |
| | spinach salad: |
| | 2 cups spinach |
| | 1/2 cup mushrooms |

|            | 2 breadsticks |
| Vegetables | 3 stalks broccoli |
| Dessert | 1/2 cup sugar-free ice cream, vanilla |

### *Friday (Total—1480 Calories)*

### BREAKFAST (174 Calories)
| | |
|---|---|
| Fruit | 1/2 cup mango (or fruit of your choice) |
| Main Dish | 2 tbsp granola layered with 1/2 cup plain nonfat yogurt |

### SNACK (214 Calories)
| | |
|---|---|
| Vegetables | 3 stalks broccoli |
| Grains | 1 granola bar, fat free |
| Dairy/Calcium | 1/4 cup fat-free ricotta cheese |

### LUNCH (391 Calories)
| | |
|---|---|
| Fruit | 1 medium apple |
| Main Dish | 1 cup black bean soup with 1 tbsp plain yogurt |
| | 1/4 cup salsa |
| | 15 baked tortilla chips |
| Dairy/Calcium | 1 packet hot cocoa, artificially sweetened |
| | 1/4 cup fat-free ricotta cheese |

### SNACK (214 Calories)
| | |
|---|---|
| Vegetables | 3 stalks broccoli |
| Grains | 1 granola bar, fat free |
| Dairy/Calcium | 1/4 cup fat-free ricotta cheese |

### DINNER (487 Calories)
| | |
|---|---|
| Main Dish | 1 chicken enchilada frozen dinner |
| | 1 cup gazpacho (or vegetable soup) |
| Vegetables | 1/2 cup coleslaw |
| Dessert | 1/2 cup fat-free pudding |

## Saturday (Total—1368 Calories)

### BREAKFAST (146 Calories)
| | |
|---|---|
| Fruit | 1 medium plum |
| Main Dish | 2 tbsp Grapenuts cereal layered with 1/2 cup fruit yogurt |

### SNACK (179 Calories)
| | |
|---|---|
| Vegetables | 1/2 cucumber |
| Grains | 4 squares graham crackers |
| Dairy/Calcium | 1/4 cup lowfat cottage cheese, calcium fortified |

### LUNCH (385 Calories)
| | |
|---|---|
| Fruit | 1 nectarine |
| Main Dish | Chicken Caesar salad: |
| | 2 oz chicken breast |
| | 2 cups romaine lettuce |
| | 1/2 medium tomato |
| | 2 tbsp croutons |
| | 1 small sourdough roll |
| Dairy/Calcium | 1/2 cup nonfat yogurt, artificially sweetened |
| | 1/4 cup lowfat cottage cheese, calcium fortified |

### SNACK (179 Calories)
| | |
|---|---|
| Vegetables | 1/2 cucumber |
| Grains | 4 squares graham crackers |
| Dairy/Calcium | 1/4 cup lowfat cottage cheese, calcium fortified |

### DINNER (479 Calories)
| | |
|---|---|
| Main Dish | 1 chicken teriyaki frozen dinner |
| | 1 cup chicken noodle soup |
| | 1 cup steamed broccoli |
| Vegetables | 1 cup tossed salad with nonfat dressing |
| Dessert | 1 thin slice pound cake |

### Sunday (Total—1359 Calories)

#### BREAKFAST (163 Calories)

| | |
|---|---|
| Fruit | 1 medium peach |
| Main Dish | 1 slice wheat toast with 1 slice (2/3 oz) melted reduced-fat cheddar |

#### SNACK (184 Calories)

| | |
|---|---|
| Vegetables | 7 florets cauliflower |
| Grains | 4 gingersnaps |
| Dairy/Calcium | 1 oz fat-free cheddar cheese |

#### LUNCH (374 Calories)

| | |
|---|---|
| Fruit | 1/2 cup peaches, canned in juice |
| Main Dish | 2 oz grilled steak with 1/2 a pepper and 1/2 cup white rice |
| Dairy/Calcium | 1/2 cup lowfat milk |
| | 1 oz fat-free cheddar cheese |

#### SNACK (184 Calories)

| | |
|---|---|
| Vegetables | 7 florets cauliflower |
| Grains | 4 gingersnaps |
| Dairy/Calcium | 1 oz fat-free cheddar cheese |

#### DINNER (454 Calories)

| | |
|---|---|
| Main Dish | 1 cheese ravioli parmigiana entrée |
| | 1/2 cup sautéed spinach with garlic |
| Vegetables | 1 cup lettuce with nonfat dressing |
| Dessert | 1 small brownie |

---

# WEEK 2

### Monday (Total—1344 Calories)

#### BREAKFAST (178 Calories)

| | |
|---|---|
| Fruit | 2 tbsp raisins |
| Main Dish | 1/2 cup oatmeal with 1/2 cup lowfat or skim milk |

## SNACK *(174 Calories)*

| | |
|---|---|
| Vegetable | 4 slices tomato |
| Grain | 1 granola bar, regular |
| Dairy/Calcium | 1 packet hot cocoa, artificially sweetened |

## LUNCH *(374 Calories)*

| | |
|---|---|
| Fruit | 1/2 medium banana |
| Main Dish | 1/2 medium pita bread stuffed with 1/4 cup hummus, lettuce, and tomato |
| Dairy/Calcium | 1 packet hot cocoa, artificially sweetened |
| | 1/4 cup fat-free ricotta cheese |

## SNACK *(177 Calories)*

| | |
|---|---|
| Vegetable | 4 slices tomato |
| Grain | 1 granola bar, regular |
| Dairy/Calcium | 1 packet hot cocoa, artificially sweetened |

## DINNER *(441 Calories)*

| | |
|---|---|
| Main Dish | 1 beef pepper steak frozen entrée |
| | Spinach salad: |
| | 2 cups spinach |
| | 1/2 cup mushrooms |
| | 2 breadsticks |
| Vegetable | 3 stalks broccoli |
| Dessert | 1/2 cup sugar-free ice cream, vanilla |

### *Tuseday (Total—1293 Calories)*

## BREAKFAST *(174 Calories)*

| | |
|---|---|
| Fruit | 1/2 cup mango |
| Main Dish | 2 tbsp granola layered with 1/2 cup plain nonfat yogurt |

## SNACK *(214 Calories)*

| | |
|---|---|
| Vegetable | 3 stalks broccoli |
| Grain | 1 granola bar, fat free |
| Dairy/Calcium | 1/4 cup fat-free ricotta cheese |

## LUNCH *(397 Calories)*

| | |
|---|---|
| Fruit | 1 medium apple |

| | |
|---|---|
| Main Dish | 1 cup black bean soup with 1 tbsp plain yogurt |
| | 1/4 cup salsa |
| | 15 baked tortilla chips |
| Dairy/Calcium | 1 packet hot cocoa, artificially sweetened |
| | 1/4 cup fat-free ricotta cheese |

### SNACK (214 Calories)

| | |
|---|---|
| Vegetable | 3 stalks broccoli |
| Grain | 1 granola bar, fat free |
| Dairy/Calcium | 1/4 cup fat-free ricotta cheese |

### DINNER (487 Calories)

| | |
|---|---|
| Main Dish | 1 chicken enchilada frozen dinner |
| | 1 cup gazpacho |
| Vegetable | 1/2 cup coleslaw |
| Dessert | 1/2 cup fat-free pudding |

### Wednesday (Total—1368 Calories)

### BREAKFAST (146 Calories)

| | |
|---|---|
| Fruit | 1 medium plum |
| Main Dish | 2 tbsp grapenuts cereal layered with 1/2 cup sugar-free yogurt |

### SNACK (179 Calories)

| | |
|---|---|
| Vegetable | 1/2 cucumber |
| Grain | 4 squares graham crackers |
| Dairy/Calcium | 1/4 cup lowfat cottage cheese, calcium fortified |

### LUNCH (385 Calories)

| | |
|---|---|
| Fruit | 1 nectarine |
| Main Dish | Chicken Caesar salad: |
| | 2 oz chicken breast |
| | 2 cups romaine lettuce |
| | 1/2 medium tomato |
| | 2 tbsp croutons |
| | 1 small sourdough roll |

| Dairy/Calcium | 1/2 cup nonfat yogurt, artificially sweetened |
| | 1/4 cup lowfat cottage cheese, calcium fortified |

### SNACK *(179 Calories)*

| Vegetable | 1/2 cucumber |
| Grain | 4 squares graham crackers |
| Dairy/Calcium | 1/4 cup lowfat cottage cheese, calcium fortified |

### DINNER *(479 Calories)*

| Main Dish | 1 chicken teriyaki frozen dinner |
| | 1 cup miso soup |
| | 1 cup Steamed broccoli |
| Vegetable | 1 cup tossed salad |
| Dessert | 1 thin slice pound cake |

### Thursday *(Total—1350 Calories)*

### BREAKFAST *(163 Calories)*

| Fruit | 1 medium peach |
| Main Dish | 1 slice wheat toast with 1 slice (2/3 oz) melted reduced fat cheddar |

### SNACK *(184 Calories)*

| Vegetable | 7 florets cauliflower |
| Grain | 4 gingersnaps |
| Dairy/Calcium | 1 oz fat-free cheddar cheese |

### LUNCH *(365 Calories)*

| Fruit | 1/2 cup peaches, canned in juice |
| Main Dish | Grilled shrimp kebab with: |
| | 2 oz shrimp |
| | 1/2 red pepper |
| | 1/2 onion |
| | on a bed of 1/2 cup brown rice |
| Dairy/Calcium | 1/2 cup lowfat milk |
| | 1 oz fat-free cheddar cheese |

*SNACK (184 Calories)*

| | |
|---|---|
| Vegetable | 7 florets cauliflower |
| Grain | 4 gingersnaps |
| Dairy/Calcium | 1 oz fat-free cheddar cheese |

*DINNER (454 Calories)*

| | |
|---|---|
| Main Dish | 1 cheese ravioli parmigiana entrée |
| | 1/2 cup sautéed spinach with garlic |
| Vegetable | 1 cup lettuce |
| Dessert | 1 small brownie |

### Friday (Total—1349 Calories)

*BREAKFAST (174 Calories)*

| | |
|---|---|
| Fruit | 1 cup cantaloupe |
| Main Dish | 1/2 cup bran flakes with 1/2 cup lowfat or skim milk |

*SNACK (170 Calories)*

| | |
|---|---|
| Vegetable | 1 carrot |
| Grain | 1 small (1 oz) whole grain roll |
| Dairy/Calcium | 1/2 cup nonfat plain yogurt |

*LUNCH (395 Calories)*

| | |
|---|---|
| Fruit | 1 cup cranberry juice, artificially sweetened |
| Main Dish | 2 oz turkey breast and 1/2 oz lowfat Swiss cheese on a 1/2 a small bagel with lettuce and tomato |
| | 1/2 cup coleslaw |
| Dairy/Calcium | 1/2 cup nonfat plain yogurt |
| | 1/2 cup orange juice, calcium fortified |

*SNACK (170 Calories)*

| | |
|---|---|
| Vegetable | 1 carrot |
| Grain | 1 small (1 oz) whole grain roll |
| Dairy/Calcium | 1/2 cup nonfat plain yogurt |

*DINNER (440 Calories)*

| | |
|---|---|
| Main Dish | 2 oz grilled salmon |

|              | 1 cup brown rice |
|              | 1 cup steamed carrots |
| Vegetable    | 1 whole dill pickle |
| Dessert      | 1/2 cup frozen yogurt, nonfat |

### Saturday (Total—1318 Calories)

**BREAKFAST (166 Calories)**

| Fruit      | 3/4 cup honeydew |
| Main Dish  | 1/2 cup oat rings with 1/2 cup lowfat or skim milk |

**SNACK (142 Calories)**

| Vegetable      | 1 stalk celery |
| Grain          | 1 small (1 oz) dinner roll |
| Dairy/Calcium  | 1/2 cup lowfat milk |

**LUNCH (384 Calories)**

| Fruit          | 1/2 cup fruit salad |
| Main Dish      | 2 oz tuna, mixed with 2 tsp lowfat mayo on 1 slice whole wheat bread |
|                | 1/2 cup three bean salad |
| Dairy/Calcium  | 1/2 cup lowfat milk |
|                | 1 oz fat-free cheddar cheese |

**SNACK (142 Calories)**

| Vegetable      | 1 stalk celery |
| Grain          | 1 small (1 oz) dinner roll |
| Dairy/Calcium  | 1/2 cup lowfat milk |

**DINNER (484 Calories)**

| Main Dish   | Spaghetti and meat sauce: |
|             | 2 oz cooked ground turkey |
|             | 1/4 cup spaghetti sauce |
|             | 3/4 cup cooked spaghetti |
|             | 1/2 cup steamed broccoli |
| Vegetable   | 7 florets cauliflower |
| Dessert     | 1/2 cup frozen yogurt, lowfat |

## Sunday (Total—1343 Calories)

### BREAKFAST (160 Calories)
| | |
|---|---|
| Fruit | 1 cup strawberries |
| Main Dish | 3/4 cup crispy rice cereal with 1/2 cup lowfat or skim milk |

### SNACK (160 Calories)
| | |
|---|---|
| Vegetable | 1/2 red pepper, sliced |
| Grain | 3 breadsticks |
| Dairy/Calcium | 1/2 cup nonfat yogurt, artificially sweetened |

### LUNCH (405 Calories)
| | |
|---|---|
| Fruit | 1 orange |
| Main Dish | 2 oz lean roast beef on a small whole wheat roll with tomato |
| | 6 oz Minestrone soup |
| Dairy/Calcium | 1/2 cup nonfat yogurt, artificially sweetened |
| | 1/4 cup lowfat cottage cheese, calcium fortified |

### SNACK (160 Calories)
| | |
|---|---|
| Vegetable | 1/2 red pepper, sliced |
| Grain | 3 breadsticks |
| Dairy/Calcium | 1/2 cup nonfat yogurt, artificially sweetened |

### DINNER (458 Calories)
| | |
|---|---|
| Main Dish | Stir-fried chicken with broccoli: |
| | 1/2 cup chicken |
| | 1/2 cup broccoli |
| | 1/2 cup carrots |
| | 1/2 cup snow peas |
| | 3/4 cup cooked brown rice |
| Vegetable | 1/2 cucumber |
| Dessert | 1/2 cup light ice cream, vanilla (or frozen yogurt) |

# WEEK 3

## *Monday (Total—1347 Calories)*

**BREAKFAST *(178 Calories)***
Fruit                2 tbsp raisins
Main Dish            1/2 cup oatmeal with 1/2 cup lowfat or skim
                     milk

**SNACK *(177 Calories)***
Vegetable            4 slices tomato'
Grain                1 granola bar, regular
Dairy/Calcium        1 packet hot cocoa, artificially sweetened

**LUNCH *(374 Calories)***
Fruit                1/2 medium banana
Main Dish            1/2 medium Pita stuffed with 1/4 cup hummus
                     lettuce and tomato
Dairy/Calcium        1 packet hot cocoa, artificially sweetened
                     1/4 cup fat-free ricotta cheese

**SNACK *(177 Calories)***
Vegetable            4 slices tomato
Grain                1 granola bar, regular
Dairy/Calcium        1 packet hot cocoa, artificially sweetened

**DINNER *(441 Calories)***
Main Dish            1 beef pepper steak frozen entrée
                     Spinach salad:
                     2 cups spinach
                     1/2 cup mushrooms
                     2 breadsticks
Vegetable            3 stalks broccoli
Dessert              1/2 cup sugar-free ice cream, vanilla

## *Tuesday (Total—1480 Calories)*
**BREAKFAST *(174 Calories)***
Fruit                1/2 cup mango

| | |
|---|---|
| Main Dish | 2 tbsp granola layered with 1/2 cup plain nonfat yogurt |

### SNACK (214 Calories)

| | |
|---|---|
| Vegetable | 3 stalks broccoli |
| Grain | 1 granola bar, fat free |
| Dairy/Calcium | 1/4 cup fat-free ricotta cheese |

### LUNCH (391 Calories)

| | |
|---|---|
| Fruit | 1 medium apple |
| Main Dish | 1 cup Black bean soup with 1 tbsp plain yogurt |
| | 1/4 cup salsa |
| | 15 baked tortilla chips |
| Dairy/Calcium | 1 packet hot cocoa, artificially sweetened |
| | 1/4 cup fat-free ricotta cheese |

### SNACK (214 Calories)

| | |
|---|---|
| Vegetable | 3 stalks broccoli |
| Grain | 1 granola bar, fat free |
| Dairy/Calcium | 1/4 cup fat-free ricotta cheese |

### DINNER (487 Calories)

| | |
|---|---|
| Main Dish | 1 chicken enchilada frozen dinner |
| | 1 cup gazpacho |
| Vegetable | 1/2 cup coleslaw |
| Dessert | 1/2 cup fat-free pudding |

### Wednesday (Total—1368 Calories)

### BREAKFAST (146 Calories)

| | |
|---|---|
| Fruit | 1 medium plum |
| Main Dish | 2 tbsp grapenuts cereal layered with 1/2 cup sugar-free yogurt |

### SNACK (179 Calories)

| | |
|---|---|
| Vegetable | 1/2 cucumber |
| Grain | 4 squares graham crackers |
| Dairy/Calcium | 1/4 cup lowfat cottage cheese, calcium fortified |

*LUNCH (385 Calories)*

| | |
|---|---|
| Fruit | 1 nectarine |
| Main Dish | Chicken Caesar salad: |
| | 2 oz chicken breast |
| | 2 cups romaine lettuce |
| | 1/2 medium tomato |
| | 2 tbsp croutons |
| | 1 small sourdough roll |
| Dairy/Calcium | 1/2 cup nonfat yogurt, artificially sweetened |
| | 1/4 cup lowfat cottage cheese, calcium fortified |

*SNACK (179 Calories)*

| | |
|---|---|
| Vegetable | 1/2 cucumber |
| Grain | 4 squares graham crackers |
| Dairy/Calcium | 1/4 cup lowfat cottage cheese, calcium fortified |

*DINNER (479 Calories)*

| | |
|---|---|
| Main Dish | 1 chicken teriyaki frozen dinner |
| | 1 cup miso soup |
| | 1 cup steamed broccoli |
| Vegetable | 1 cup tossed salad |
| Dessert | 1 thin slice pound cake |

### *Thursday (Total—1153 Calories)*

*BREAKFAST (166 Calories)*

| | |
|---|---|
| Fruit | 1 medium peach |
| Main Dish | 1 slice wheat toast with 1 slice (2/3 oz) melted reduced fat cheddar |

*SNACK (184 Calories)*

| | |
|---|---|
| Vegetable | 7 florets cauliflower |
| Grain | 4 gingersnaps |
| Dairy/Calcium | 1 oz fat-free cheddar cheese |

*LUNCH (165 Calories)*

| | |
|---|---|
| Fruit | 1/2 cup peaches, canned in juice |

| Main Dish | Grilled shrimp kebab with: |
|---|---|
| | 2 oz shrimp |
| | 1/2 red pepper |
| | 1/2 onion |
| | on a bed of 1/2 cup brown rice |
| Dairy/Calcium | 1/2 cup lowfat milk |
| | 1 oz fat-free cheddar cheese |

### SNACK (184 Calories)

| Vegetable | 7 florets cauliflower |
|---|---|
| Grain | 4 gingersnaps |
| Dairy/Calcium | 1 oz fat-free cheddar cheese |

### DINNER (454 Calories)

| Main Dish | 1 cheese ravioli parmigiana entrée |
|---|---|
| | 1/2 cup sautéed spinach with garlic |
| Vegetable | 1 cup lettuce |
| Dessert | 1 small brownie |

### Friday (Total—1349 Calories)

### BREAKFAST (174 Calories)

| Fruit | 1 cup cantaloupe |
|---|---|
| Main Dish | 1/2 cup bran flakes with 1/2 cup lowfat or skim milk |

### SNACK (170 Calories)

| Vegetable | 1 carrot |
|---|---|
| Grain | 1 small (1 oz) whole grain roll |
| Dairy/Calcium | 1/2 cup nonfat plain yogurt |

### LUNCH (395 Calories)

| Fruit | 1 cup cranberry juice, artificially sweetened |
|---|---|
| Main Dish | 2 oz turkey breast and 1/2 oz lowfat Swiss cheese on 1/2 a small bagel with lettuce and tomato |
| | 1/2 cup coleslaw |
| Dairy/Calcium | 1/2 cup nonfat plain yogurt |
| | 1/2 cup orange juice, calcium fortified |

### SNACK *(170 Calories)*

| | |
|---|---|
| Vegetable | 1 carrot |
| Grain | 1 small (1 oz) whole grain roll |
| Dairy/Calcium | 1/2 cup nonfat plain yogurt |

### DINNER *(440 Calories)*

| | |
|---|---|
| Main Dish | 2 oz grilled salmon |
| | 1 cup brown rice |
| | 1 cup steamed carrots |
| Vegetable | 1 whole dill pickle |
| Dessert | 1/2 cup frozen yogurt, nonfat |

### Saturday *(Total—1318 Calories)*

### BREAKFAST *(166 Calories)*

| | |
|---|---|
| Fruit | 3/4 cup honeydew |
| Main Dish | 1/2 cup oat rings with 1/2 cup lowfat or skim milk |

### SNACK *(142 Calories)*

| | |
|---|---|
| Vegetable | 1 stalk celery |
| Grain | 1 small (1 oz) dinner roll |
| Dairy/Calcium | 1/2 cup lowfat milk |

### LUNCH *(384 Calories)*

| | |
|---|---|
| Fruit | 1/2 cup fruit salad |
| Main Dish | 2 oz tuna, mixed with 2 tsp lowfat mayo on 1 slice whole wheat bread |
| | 1/2 cup three-bean salad |
| Dairy/Calcium | 1/2 cup lowfat milk |
| | 1 oz fat-free cheddar cheese |

### SNACK *(142 Calories)*

| | |
|---|---|
| Vegetable | 1 stalk celery |
| Grain | 1 small (1 oz) dinner roll |
| Dairy/Calcium | 1/2 cup lowfat milk |

### DINNER *(484 Calories)*

| | |
|---|---|
| Main Dish | Spaghetti and meat sauce: |
| | 2 oz cooked ground turkey |

|                | 1/4 cup spaghetti sauce |
|----------------|-------------------------|
|                | 3/4 cup cooked spaghetti |
|                | 1/2 cup steamed broccoli |
| Vegetable      | 7 florets cauliflower |
| Dessert        | 1/2 cup frozen yogurt, lowfat |

### Sunday (Total—1343 Calories)

### BREAKFAST (160 Calories)
| Fruit     | 1 cup strawberries |
|-----------|--------------------|
| Main Dish | 3/4 cup crispy rice cereal with 1/2 cup lowfat or skim milk |

### SNACK (160 Calories)
| Vegetable      | 1/2 red pepper, sliced |
|----------------|------------------------|
| Grain          | 3 breadsticks |
| Dairy/Calcium  | 1/2 cup nonfat yogurt, artificially sweetened |

### LUNCH (405 Calories)
| Fruit          | 1 orange |
|----------------|----------|
| Main Dish      | 2 oz lean roast beef on a small whole wheat roll with tomato |
|                | 6 oz minestrone soup |
| Dairy/Calcium  | 1/2 cup nonfat yogurt, artificially sweetened |
|                | 1/4 cup lowfat cottage cheese, calcium fortified |

### SNACK (160 Calories)
| Vegetable      | 1/2 red pepper, sliced |
|----------------|------------------------|
| Grain          | 3 breadsticks |
| Dairy/Calcium  | 1/2 cup nonfat yogurt, artificially sweetened |

### DINNER (458 Calories)
| Main | Stir-fried chicken with broccoli: |
|------|-----------------------------------|
|      | 1/2 cup chicken |
|      | 1/2 cup broccoli |
|      | 1/2 cup carrots |
|      | 1/2 cup snow peas |
|      | 3/4 cup cooked brown rice |

| Vegetable | 1/2 cucumber |
| Dessert | 1/2 cup light ice cream, vanilla |

---

# WEEK 4

### *Monday (Total—1170 Calories)*

**BREAKFAST (178 Calories)**

| Fruit | 2 tbsp raisins |
| Main Dish | 1/2 cup oatmeal with 1/2 cup lowfat or skim milk |

**SNACK ( Calories)**

| Vegetable | 4 slices tomato |
| Grain | 1 granola bar, regular |
| Dairy/Calcium | 1 packet hot cocoa, artificially sweetened |

**LUNCH (374 Calories)**

| Fruit | 1/2 medium banana |
| Main Dish | 1/2 medium pita bread stuffed with 1/4 cup hummus, lettuce, and tomato |
| Dairy/Calcium | 1 packet hot cocoa, artificially sweetened |
| | 1/4 cup fat-free ricotta cheese |

**SNACK (177 Calories)**

| Vegetable | 4 slices tomato |
| Grain | 1 granola bar, regular |
| Dairy/Calcium | 1 packet hot cocoa, artificially sweetened |

**DINNER (441 Calories)**

| Main Dish | 1 beef pepper steak frozen entrée |
| | Spinach salad: |
| | 2 cups spinach |
| | 1/2 cup mushrooms |
| | 2 breadsticks |
| Vegetable | 3 stalks broccoli |
| Dessert | 1/2 cup sugar-free ice cream, vanilla |

### Tuesday (Total—1480 Calories)

**BREAKFAST (174 Calories)**

| | |
|---|---|
| Fruit | 1/2 cup mango |
| Main Dish | 2 tbsp granola layered with 1/2 cup plain nonfat yogurt |

**SNACK (214 Calories)**

| | |
|---|---|
| Vegetable | 3 stalks broccoli |
| Grain | 1 granola bar, fat free |
| Dairy/Calcium | 1/4 cup fat-free ricotta cheese |

**LUNCH (391 Calories)**

| | |
|---|---|
| Fruit | 1 medium apple |
| Main Dish | 1 cup black bean soup with 1 tbsp plain yogurt |
| | 1/4 cup salsa |
| | 15 baked tortilla chips |
| Dairy/Calcium | 1 packet hot cocoa, artificially sweetened |
| | 1/4 cup fat-free ricotta cheese |

**SNACK (214 Calories)**

| | |
|---|---|
| Vegetable | 3 stalks broccoli |
| Grain | 1 granola bar, fat free |
| Dairy/Calcium | 1/4 cup fat-free ricotta cheese |

**DINNER (487 Calories)**

| | |
|---|---|
| Main Dish | 1 chicken enchilada frozen dinner |
| | 1 cup gazpacho |
| Vegetable | 1/2 cup coleslaw |
| Dessert | 1/2 cup fat-free pudding |

### Wednesday (Total—1368 Calories)

**BREAKFAST (146 Calories)**

| | |
|---|---|
| Fruit | 1 medium plum |
| Main Dish | 2 tbsp grapenuts cereal layered with 1/2 cup sugar-free yogurt |

## SNACK *(179 Calories)*

| | |
|---|---|
| Vegetable | 1/2 cucumber |
| Grain | 4 squares graham crackers |
| Dairy/Calcium | 1/4 cup lowfat cottage cheese, calcium fortified |

## LUNCH *(385 Calories)*

| | |
|---|---|
| Fruit | 1 nectarine |
| Main Dish | Chicken Caesar salad: |
| | 2 oz chicken breast |
| | 2 cups romaine lettuce |
| | 1/2 medium tomato |
| | 2 tbsp croutons |
| | 1 small sourdough roll |
| Dairy/Calcium | 1/2 cup nonfat yogurt, artificially sweetened |
| | 1/4 cup lowfat cottage cheese, calcium fortified |

## SNACK *(179 Calories)*

| | |
|---|---|
| Vegetable | 1/2 cucumber |
| Grain | 4 squares graham crackers |
| Dairy/Calcium | 1/4 cup lowfat cottage cheese, calcium fortified |

## DINNER *(479 Calories)*

| | |
|---|---|
| Main Dish | 1 chicken teriyaki frozen dinner |
| | 1 cup miso soup |
| | 1 cup steamed broccoli |
| Vegetable | 1 cup tossed salad |
| Dessert | 1 thin slice pound cake |

### Thursday *(Total—1350 Calories)*

## BREAKFAST *(163 Calories)*

| | |
|---|---|
| Fruit | 1 medium peach |
| Main Dish | 1 slice wheat toast with 1 slice (2/3 oz) melted reduced-fat cheddar |

### SNACK *(184 Calories)*

| | |
|---|---|
| Vegetable | 7 florets cauliflower |
| Grain | 4 gingersnaps |
| Dairy/Calcium | 1 oz fat-free cheddar cheese |

### LUNCH *(365 Calories)*

| | |
|---|---|
| Fruit | 1/2 cup peaches, canned in juice |
| Main Dish | Grilled shrimp kebab with: |
| | 2 oz shrimp |
| | 1/2 red pepper |
| | 1/2 onion on a bed of 1/2 cup brown rice |
| Dairy/Calcium | 1/2 cup lowfat milk |
| | 1 oz fat-free cheddar cheese |

### SNACK *(184 Calories)*

| | |
|---|---|
| Vegetable | 7 florets cauliflower |
| Grain | 4 gingersnaps |
| Dairy/Calcium | 1 oz fat-free cheddar cheese |

### DINNER *(454 Calories)*

| | |
|---|---|
| Main Dish | 1 cheese ravioli parmigiana entrée |
| | 1/2 cup sautéed spinach with garlic |
| Vegetable | 1 cup lettuce |
| Dessert | 1 small brownie |

### *Friday (Total—1349 Calories)*

### BREAKFAST *(174 Calories)*

| | |
|---|---|
| Fruit | 1 cup cantaloupe |
| Main Dish | 1/2 cup bran flakes with 1/2 cup lowfat or skim milk |

### SNACK *(170 Calories)*

| | |
|---|---|
| Vegetable | 1 carrot |
| Grain | 1 small (1 oz) whole grain roll |
| Dairy/Calcium | 1/2 cup nonfat plain yogurt |

### LUNCH *(395 Calories)*

| | |
|---|---|
| Fruit | 1 cup cranberry juice, artificially sweetened |

| | |
|---|---|
| Main Dish | 2 oz turkey breast and 1/2 oz lowfat Swiss cheese on 1/2 a small bagel with lettuce and tomato |
| | 1/2 cup cole slaw |
| Dairy/Calcium | 1/2 cup nonfat plain yogurt |
| | 1/2 cup orange juice, calcium fortified |

### SNACK *(170 Calories)*

| | |
|---|---|
| Vegetable | 1 carrot |
| Grain | 1 small (1 oz) whole grain roll |
| Dairy/Calcium | 1/2 cup nonfat plain yogurt |

### DINNER *(440 Calories)*

| | |
|---|---|
| Main Dish | 2 oz grilled salmon |
| | 1 cup brown rice |
| | 1 cup steamed carrots |
| Vegetable | 1 whole dill pickle |
| Dessert | 1/2 cup frozen yogurt, nonfat |

## Saturday *(Total—1318 Calories)*

### BREAKFAST *(166 Calories)*

| | |
|---|---|
| Fruit | 3/4 cup honeydew |
| Main Dish | 1/2 cup oat rings with 1/2 cup lowfat or skim milk |

### SNACK *(142 Calories)*

| | |
|---|---|
| Vegetable | 1 stalk celery |
| Grain | 1 small (1 oz) dinner roll |
| Dairy/Calcium | 1/2 cup lowfat milk |

### LUNCH *(384 Calories)*

| | |
|---|---|
| Fruit | 1/2 cup fruit salad |
| Main Dish | 2 oz tuna, mixed with 2 tsp lowfat mayo on 1 slice whole wheat bread |
| | 1/2 cup three-bean salad |
| Dairy/Calcium | 1/2 cup lowfat milk |
| | 1 oz fat-free cheddar cheese |

*SNACK (142 Calories)*

| | |
|---|---|
| Vegetable | 1 stalk celery |
| Grain | 1 small (1 oz) dinner roll |
| Dairy/Calcium | 1/2 cup lowfat milk |

*DINNER (484 Calories)*

| | |
|---|---|
| Main Dish | Spaghetti and meat sauce: |
| | 2 oz cooked ground turkey |
| | 1/4 cup spaghetti sauce |
| | 3/4 cup cooked spaghetti |
| | 1/2 cup steamed broccoli |
| Vegetable | 7 florets cauliflower |
| Dessert | 1/2 cup frozen yogurt, lowfat |

### *Sunday (Total—1343 Calories)*

*BREAKFAST (160 Calories)*

| | |
|---|---|
| Fruit | 1 cup strawberries |
| Main Dish | 3/4 cup crispy rice cereal with 1/2 cup lowfat or skim milk |

*SNACK (160 Calories)*

| | |
|---|---|
| Vegetable | 1/2 red pepper, sliced |
| Grain | 3 breadsticks |
| Dairy/Calcium | 1/2 cup nonfat yogurt, artificially sweetened |

*LUNCH (405 Calories)*

| | |
|---|---|
| Fruit | 1 orange |
| Main Dish | 2 oz lean roast beef on a small whole wheat roll with tomato |
| | 6 oz minestrone soup |
| Dairy/Calcium | 1/2 cup nonfat yogurt, artificially sweetened |
| | 1/4 cup lowfat cottage cheese, calcium fortified |

*SNACK (160 Calories)*

| | |
|---|---|
| Vegetable | 1/2 red pepper, sliced |
| Grain | 3 breadsticks |
| Dairy/Calcium | 1/2 cup nonfat yogurt, artificially sweetened |

*DINNER (458 Calories)*

| | |
|---|---|
| Main Dish | Stir-fried chicken with broccoli: |
| | 1/2 cup chicken |
| | 1/2 cup broccoli |
| | 1/2 cup carrots |
| | 1/2 cup snow peas |
| | 3/4 cup cooked brown rice |
| Vegetable | 1/2 cucumber |
| Dessert | 1/2 cup light ice cream, vanilla (or frozen yogurt) |

---

# SAMPLE WEEKLY MENUS:
## 1200 AND 1500 CALORIES PER DAY

### *Sample Weekly Diet—Approximately 1200 calories per day*

| | breakfast | lunch | snack | dinner |
|---|---|---|---|---|
| DAY 1 | morning breakfast shake | turkeyburgers southwestern style celery and carrot sticks | 1 orange | pasta and eggplant Provençal salad pears in red wine |
| DAY 2 | oatmeal and raisins | green pea soup citrus salad sourdough roll | 1 banana | ginger-sesame salmon brown rice pilaf steamed broccoli peach frozen yogurt |
| DAY 3 | 3/4 cup bran flakes 1 cup skim milk | gazpacho chef's salad 2 ginger cookies | 1 fresh apple | vegetarian stew green salad with |

|  |  |  |  |
|---|---|---|---|
| | 1/2 cup fresh blueberries | | | cucumber and yogurt dressing peach crumble |
| DAY 4 | 1 cup muesli cereal 1/2 cup skim milk 1/2 fresh grapefruit | tomato soup 1 whole wheat dinner roll tabbouleh salad | 2 dried apricot halves | beef bourguignon brussels sprouts and chestnuts brown rice lemon sherbet |
| DAY 5 | fruit and yogurt shake | chicken soup carrot and raisin salad 1 whole wheat dinner roll | 1 banana | Mexican bean pie green salad with spicy yogurt dressing apple crisp |
| DAY 6 | herbal all-bran shake | grilled tuna warm coriander sauce garlic mashed potatoes French peas fresh fruit salad | 1 orange | stir-fry vegetables and rice pineapple meringue pie |
| DAY 7 | 1/2 fresh grapefruit 1 slice whole grain wheat toast 1 teaspoon butter | 3 bean Mexican salad fresh peaches in lemon juice | 1 plum | chicken with tarragon glazed carrots mixed berry sherbet |

### Sample Weekly Diet—1500 calories per day

|  | breakfast | lunch | snack | dinner |
|---|---|---|---|---|
| DAY 1 | nonfat yogurt shake 1 fresh pear | macaroni and cheese green salad with vinaigrette dressing 1 whole wheat dinner roll | 2 dried apricot halves | whitefish with ginger and lemon glazed carrots mixed berry sherbet 1 chocolate chip cookie |
| DAY 2 | banana fruit shake | gazpacho lentil patty with cucumber and yogurt dressing sourdough roll | 1 orange | mushrooms à la grecque turkey breast in white wine sauce garlic mashed potatoes apple crisp nonfat whipped cream |
| DAY 3 | oatmeal and raisins 1 orange or banana | spicy bean chili celery and carrot sticks 1 banana | 1 slice zucchini bread | oven-baked sesame chicken green salad with lemon tahini dressing peach crumble |
| DAY 4 | 1 cup shredded wheat | chicken and okra gumbo Greek salad | 1 banana | bruschetta spaghetti with |

| | Breakfast | Lunch | Snack | Dinner |
|---|---|---|---|---|
| | 1 cup skim milk 1/2 cup strawberries or blueberries | | | artichoke hearts green salad with vinaigrette dressing 1 ginger cookie |
| DAY 5 | 1 cup of muesli 1/2 cup of skim milk | grilled chicken breast sandwich carrot and celery sticks | 1 apple | spinach, brown rice and tofu green salad with oriental dressing key lime pie |
| DAY 6 | fat-free yogurt shake with strawberries | salmon and scallops brochettes green salad with oriental dressing | 1 orange | navy bean stew 1 slice soda bread 2 apricot almond squares |
| DAY 7 | oatmeal and raisins 1 small orange | tuna sandwich on rye carrot and celery sticks 2 ginger cookies | 1 apple | minestrone chicken cacciatore green salad with vinaigrette dressing 1 whole wheat dinner roll peach frozen yogurt |

EXCHANGE LIST MENU PLANS

# DAILY MEAL PLANS FROM 1200 TO 2500 CALORIES USING AN EXCHANGE LIST

The following menus have from 1200 calories to 2500 calories—about 55 to 58 percent from carbohydrates, 19 to 23 percent from proteins, and 19 to 24 percent from fats. There are three different plans in each calorie group depending on your daily milk and dairy intake. Each day, plan your meals using the suggested servings from each food exchange or group.

**1200-calorie daily meal plan (includes 2 cups milk) (women only)**
6 starch/bread exchanges
3 fruit exchanges
3 vegetable exchanges
2 milk/dairy exchanges (nonfat milk)
4 meat/protein exchanges (lean to medium fat)
2 fat exchanges

**1200-calorie daily meal plan (includes 1 cup milk) (women only)**
6 starch/bread exchanges
4 fruit exchanges
3 vegetable exchanges
1 milk/dairy exchange (nonfat milk)
4 meat/protein exchanges (lean to medium fat)
2 fat exchanges

**1200-calorie daily meal plan (includes no milk)(women only)**
7 starch/bread exchanges
4 fruit exchanges
2 vegetable exchanges
0 milk/dairy exchanges (nonfat milk)
5 meat/protein exchanges (lean to medium fat)
2 fat exchanges

**1350-calorie daily food plan (includes 2 milk servings)**
6 starch/bread exchanges
4 fruit exchanges
2 vegetable exchanges
2 milk/dairy exchanges (nonfat milk)
5 meat/protein exchanges (lean to medium fat)
3 fat exchanges

**1350-calorie**
**daily food plan**
**(includes 1**
**milk serving)**

7 starch/bread exchanges
4 fruit exchanges
2 vegetable exchanges
1 milk/dairy exchange (nonfat milk)
5 meat/protein exchanges (lean to medium fat)
3 fat exchanges

**1350-calorie**
**daily food plan**
**(includes 0 to 1/2**
**milk servings)**

7 starch/bread exchanges
4 fruit exchanges
3 vegetable exchanges
0 to 1/2 milk/dairy exchanges (nonfat milk)
5 meat/protein exchanges (lean to medium fat)
3 fat exchanges

**1500-calorie**
**daily food plan**
**(includes 2**
**milk servings)**

7 starch/bread exchanges
4 fruit exchanges
3 vegetable exchanges
2 milk/dairy exchanges (nonfat milk)
5 meat/protein exchanges (lean to medium fat)
4 fat exchanges

**1500-calorie**
**daily food plan**
**(includes 1**
**milk serving)**

8 starch/bread exchanges
4 fruit exchanges
2 vegetable exchanges
1 milk/dairy exchange (nonfat milk)
6 meat/protein exchanges (lean to medium fat)
3 fat exchanges

**1500-calorie**
**daily food plan**
**(includes 0**
**milk servings)**

9 starch/bread exchanges
4 fruit exchanges
3 vegetable exchanges
0 milk/dairy exchanges
6 meat/protein exchanges (lean to medium fat)
3 fat exchanges

**1700-calorie daily food plan (includes 2 milk ervings)**
- 8 starch/bread exchanges
- 5 fruit exchanges
- 3 vegetable exchanges
- 2 milk/dairy exchanges (1% milk)
- 6 meat/protein exchanges (lean to medium fat)
- 3 fat exchanges

**1700-calorie daily food plan (includes 1 milk serving)**
- 9 starch/bread exchanges
- 5 fruit exchanges
- 3 vegetable exchanges
- 1 milk/dairy exchange (1% milk)
- 6 meat/protein exchanges (lean to medium fat)
- 3 fat exchanges

**1700-calorie daily food plan (includes 0 to 1/2 milk servings)**
- 9 starch/bread exchanges
- 5 fruit exchanges
- 3 vegetable exchanges
- 0-1/2 milk/dairy exchanges (1% milk)
- 7 meat/protein exchanges (lean to medium fat)
- 3 fat exchanges

**1900-calorie daily food plan (includes 2 milk servings)**
- 9 starch/bread exchanges
- 6 fruit exchanges
- 2 vegetable exchanges
- 2 milk/dairy exchanges (1% milk)
- 7 meat/protein exchanges (lean to medium fat)
- 4 fat exchanges

**1900-calorie daily food plan (includes 1 milk serving)**
- 10 starch/bread exchanges
- 6 fruit exchanges
- 2 vegetable exchanges
- 1 milk/dairy exchange (1% milk)
- 8 meat/protein exchanges (lean to medium fat)
- 4 fat exchanges

| **1900-calorie daily food plan (includes 1/2 milk serving)** | 10 starch/bread exchanges<br>7 fruit exchanges<br>2 vegetable exchanges<br>1/2 milk/dairy exchange (1% milk)<br>7 meat/protein exchanges (lean to medium fat)<br>4 fat exchanges |
| --- | --- |
| **2100-calorie daily food plan (includes 2 1/2 milk servings)** | 10 starch/bread exchanges<br>5 fruit exchanges<br>3 vegetable exchanges<br>2 1/2 milk/dairy exchanges (1% milk)<br>8 meat/protein exchanges (lean to medium fat)<br>5 fat exchanges |
| **2100-calorie daily food plan (includes 1 milk serving)** | 11 starch/bread exchanges<br>6 fruit exchanges<br>4 vegetable exchanges<br>1 milk/dairy exchanges (1% milk)<br>8 meat/protein exchanges (lean to medium fat)<br>5 fat exchanges |
| **2100-calorie daily food plan (includes 1/2 milk serving)** | 11 starch/bread exchanges<br>6 fruit exchanges<br>4 vegetable exchanges<br>1/2 milk/dairy exchange (1% milk)<br>8 meat/protein exchanges (lean to medium fat)<br>6 fat exchanges |
| **2300-calorie daily food plan (includes 3 milk servings)** | 11 starch/bread exchanges<br>6 fruit exchanges<br>4 vegetable exchanges<br>3 milk/dairy exchanges (1% milk)<br>8 meat/protein exchanges (lean to medium fat)<br>5 fat exchanges |

**2300-calorie daily food plan (includes 1 milk serving)**

13 starch/bread exchanges
6 fruit exchanges
4 vegetable exchanges
1 milk/dairy exchange (1% milk)
7 meat/protein exchanges (lean to medium fat)
7 fat exchanges

**2300-calorie daily food plan (includes 0 milk servings)**

13 starch/bread exchanges
7 fruit exchanges
4 vegetable exchanges
0 milk/dairy exchanges
7 meat/protein exchanges (lean to medium fat)
7 fat exchanges

**2500-calorie daily food plan (includes 3 milk servings)**

12 starch/bread exchanges
7 fruit exchanges
4 vegetable exchanges
3 milk/dairy exchanges (1% milk)
8 meat/protein exchanges (lean to medium fat)
6 fat exchanges

**2500-calorie daily food plan (includes 1 milk serving)**

13 starch/bread exchanges
8 fruit exchanges
4 vegetable exchanges
1 milk/dairy exchange (1% milk)
8 meat/protein exchanges (lean to medium fat)
8 fat exchanges

**2500-calorie daily food plan (includes 0 milk servings)**

13 starch/bread exchanges
8 fruit exchanges
5 vegetable exchanges
0 milk/dairy exchanges
9 meat/protein exchanges (lean to medium fat)
8 fat exchanges

### *Starch and Bread List*

Each item in this list contains approximately 15 grams of carbohydrate, 3 grams of protein, a trace of fat, and 80 calories. Whole grain products average about 2 grams of fiber per exchange or serving. Foods in this group are a major source of thiamin, niacin, iron, fiber, and zinc. They are also a vital part of a healthy, balanced diet, and can be an aid to weight loss.

The carbohydrates in bread or starch exchanges are complex. These complex sugars cannot be absorbed from the intestinal tract in this form. These complex sugars must first be converted to simple sugars (in the intestine). Once the complex sugar is "broken down" into smaller parts, the simple sugar is absorbed. Blood sugar goes up, but much more slowly.

**Cereals/Grains/Pasta**

| | |
|---|---|
| Bran cereals, concentrated*(such as Bran Buds, All Bran) | 1/3 cup |
| Bran cereals, flaked* | 1/2 cup |
| Bulgur (cooked) | 1/2 cup |
| Cooked cereals | 1/2 cup |
| Cornmeal (dry) | 2 1/2 tbsp |
| Grapenuts | 3 tbsp |
| Grits (cooked) | 1/2 cup |
| Other ready-to-eat unsweetened cereals | 3/4 cup |
| Pasta (cooked) | 1/2 cup |
| Puffed cereal | 1 1/2 cup |
| Rice, white or brown (cooked) | 1/3 cup |
| Shredded wheat | 1/2 cup |
| Wheat germ* | 3 tbsp |

*3 grams or more of fiber per exchange.

**Dried Beans/Peas/Lentils**

| | |
|---|---|
| Beans and peas (cooked)* (such as kidney, white, split, black-eyed) | 1/3 cup |
| Lentils (cooked)* | 1/3 cup |

| | |
|---|---|
| Baked beans* | 1/4 cup |

*3 grams or more of fiber per exchange.

### Starchy Vegetables

| | |
|---|---|
| Corn* | 1/2 cup |
| Corn on cob, 6 in. long* | 1 |
| Lima beans* | 1/2 cup |
| Peas, green (canned or frozen)* | 1/2 cup |
| Plantain* | 1/2 cup |
| Potato, baked | 1 small (3 oz) |
| Potato, mashed | 1/2 cup |
| Squash, winter* (acorn, butternut) | 1 cup |
| Yam, sweet potato, plain | 1/3 cup |

*3 grams or more of fiber per exchange.

### Bread

| | |
|---|---|
| Bagel | 1/2 (1 oz |
| Bread sticks, crisp, 4 in. long x 1/2 in. | 2 (2/3 oz) |
| Croutons, lowfat | 1 cup |
| English muffin | 1/2 |
| Frankfurter or hamburger bun | 1/2 (1 oz) |
| Pita, 6 in. across | 1/2 |
| Plain roll, small | 1 (1 oz) |
| Raisin, unfrosted | 1 slice (1 oz) |
| Rye, pumpernickel | 1 slice (1 oz) |
| Tortilla, 6 in. across | 1 |
| White (including French, Italian) | 1 slice (1 oz) |
| Whole wheat | 1 slice (1 oz) |

### Crackers/Snacks

| | |
|---|---|
| Animal crackers | 8 |
| Graham crackers, 2 1/2 in. square | 3 |
| Matzoh | 3/4 oz |
| Melba toast | 5 slices |
| Oyster crackers | 24 |
| Popcorn (popped, no fat added) | 3 cups |
| Pretzels | 3/4 oz |

| | |
|---|---|
| RyKrisp, 2 in. by 3 1/2 in. | 4 |
| Saltine-type crackers | 6 |
| Whole-wheat crackers, no fat added* (crisp breads, such as Finn, Kavli, Wasa) 2–4 slices | (3/4 oz) |

*3 grams or more of fiber per exchange.

**Starch Foods Prepared with Fat**
(*count as 1 starch/bread exchange, plus 1 fat exchange*)

| | |
|---|---|
| Biscuit, 2 1/2 in. across | 1 |
| Chow mein noodles | 1/2 cup |
| Corn bread, 2 in. cube | 1 (2 oz) |
| Cracker, round butter type | 6 |
| French fried potatoes, 2 in. to 3 1/2 in. long | 10 |
| Muffin, plain, small | 1 |
| Pancake, 4 in. across | 2 |
| Stuffing, bread (prepared) | 1/4 cup |
| Taco shell, 6 in. across | 2 |
| Waffle, 4 1/2 in. square | 1 |
| Whole-wheat crackers fat added* (such as Triscuit®) | 4–6 (1 oz) |

*3 grams or more of fiber per exchange.

---

### Fruit List

Each item on this list contains about 15 grams of carbohydrate and 60 calories. Fresh, frozen, and dried fruits have about 2 grams of fiber per serving or exchange. Fruits are major sources of vitamins A and C, potassium, folic acid, soluble and insoluble fiber.

The carbohydrates in fruit exchanges are simple. When these sugars are ingested, they rapidly leave the intestinal tract and enter the bloodstream. The blood sugar goes up rapidly. Unless otherwise noted, the serving size for one fruit exchange is 1/2 cup of fresh fruit or fruit juice or 1/4 cup of dried fruit.

**Fresh, Frozen, and Unsweetened Canned Fruit**

| | |
|---|---|
| Apple (raw, 2 in across) | 1 apple |
| Applesauce (unsweetened) | 1/2 cup |

| | |
|---|---|
| Apricots (medium, raw) | 4 apricots |
| Apricots (canned) | 1/2 cup, or 4 halves |
| Banana (9 in. long) | 1/2 banana |
| Blackberries (raw)* | 3/4 cup |
| Blueberries (raw)* | 3/4 cup |
| Cantaloupe (5 in. across) (Cubes) | 1/3 melon, or 1 cup |
| Cherries (large, raw) | 12 Cherries |
| Cherries (canned) | 1/2 cup |
| Figs (raw, 2 in. across) | 2 figs |
| Fruit cocktail (canned) | 1/2 cup |
| Grapefruit (medium) | 1/2 grapefruit |
| Grapefruit (segments) | 3/4 cup |
| Grapes (small) | 15 grapes |
| Honeydew melon (medium) (cubes) | 1/8 melon, or 1 cup |
| Kiwi (large) | 1 kiwi |
| Mandarin oranges | 3/4 cup |
| Mango (small) | 1/2 mango |
| Orange (2 1/2 in. across) | 1 orange |
| Papaya | 1 cup |
| Peach (2 3/4 in. across) | 1 peach, or 3/4 cup |
| Peaches (canned) | 1/2 cup, or 2 halves |
| Pear | 1/2 large, or 1 small |
| Pears (canned) | 1/2 cup, or 2 halves |
| Persimmon (medium, native) | 2 persimmons |
| Pineapple (raw) | 3/4 cup |
| Pineapple (canned) | 1/2 cup |
| Plum (raw, 2 in. across) | 2 plums |
| Pomegranate* | 1/2 pomegranate |
| Raspberries (raw)* | 1 cup |
| Strawberries (raw, whole)* | 1 1/4 cup |

| | |
|---|---|
| Tangerine (2 1/2 in. across)* | 2 tangerines |
| Watermelon (cubes) | 1 1/4 cup |

*3 grams or more of fiber per exchange.

**Dried Fruit**

| | |
|---|---|
| Apples* | 4 rings |
| Apricots* | 7 halves |
| Dates | 2 1/2 medium |
| Figs* | 1 1/2 |
| Prunes* | 3 medium |
| Raisins | 2 tbsp |

*3 grams or more of fiber per exchange.

**Fruit Juice**

| | |
|---|---|
| Apple juice or cider | 1/2 cup |
| Cranberry juice cocktail | 1/3 cup |
| Cranberry juice cocktail, reduced calorie | 1 cup |
| Fruit juice blends, 100% juice | 1/3 cup |
| Grapefruit juice | 1/2 cup |
| Grape juice | 1/3 cup |
| Orange juice | 1/2 cup |
| Pineapple juice | 1/2 cup |
| Prune juice | 1/3 cup |

---

### *Vegetable List*

Each vegetable serving on this list contains about 5 grams of carbohydrate, 2 grams of protein, and 25 calories. Vegetables are high in certain nutrients, such as potassium, vitamins A and C, and folic acid. Vegetables contain 2 to 3 grams of dietary fiber. Unless otherwise noted, the serving size for vegetables (one vegetable exchange) is 1/2 cup of cooked vegetables or vegetable juice.

Artichoke (1/2 medium)
Asparagus
Beans (green, wax, Italian)
Bean sprouts

Beets
Broccoli
Brussels sprouts
Cabbage, cooked
Carrots
Cauliflower
Eggplant
Greens (collard, mustard, turnip)
Kohlrabi
Leeks
Mushrooms, cooked
Okra
Onions
Pea pods
Peppers (green)
Rutabaga
Sauerkraut*
Spinach, cooked
Summer squash (crookneck)
Tomato (one large)
Tomato or vegetable juice*
Turnips
Water chestnuts
Zucchini, cooked

(Starchy vegetables such as corn, peas, and potatoes are found in the Starch and Bread List. For *free vegetables—any vegetable that contains fewer than 20 calories per serving—see the* Free Foods List.)

*400 mg or more of sodium per exchange.

---

### Milk List

Each serving of milk or milk products on this list contains about 12 grams of carbohydrate and 8 grams of protein. Milk and yogurt are the body's main source of calcium, riboflavin, protein, zinc, vitamins B12 and D. Foods in this group are good for growth, strong bones, and convalescence. The sugar in a milk exchange may produce a slower rise in blood sugar. This is primarily because the protein and fat in milk reduce the rate of absorption of sugar from the intestine. The calories and amount of fat vary, depending on the percent of fat in the milk. The list is divided into three parts based on the amount of fat and calories.

**Skim and Very Lowfat Milk (trace amounts of fat and 90 calories per serving)**

| | |
|---|---|
| Skim milk | 1 cup |
| 1/2% milk | 1 cup |
| 1% milk | 1 cup |
| Lowfat or nonfat buttermilk | 1 cup |
| Evaporated skim milk | 1/2 cup |
| Dry nonfat milk | 1/3 cup dry |
| Lowfat or nonfat fruit-flavored yogurt sweetened with aspartame or with a nonnutritive sweetener | 1 cup Plain |
| 1 cup Plain nonfat yogurt | 3/4 cup |

**Lowfat Milk (5 grams of fat and 120 calories per serving)**

| | |
|---|---|
| 2% milk | 1 cup |
| Sweet acidophilus milk | 1 cup |
| Plain lowfat yogurt (with added nonfat milk solids) | 8 oz |

**Whole Milk (8 grams of fat and 150 calories per serving)**

| | |
|---|---|
| Whole milk | 1 cup |
| Evaporated whole milk | 1/2 cup |
| Whole plain yogurt | 8 oz |
| Goat's milk | 1 cup |
| Kefir | 1 cup |

---

### *Meat List*

Each serving of meat and substitutes on this list contains about 7 grams of protein and trace amounts of carbohydrate. Besides protein meat is a major source of iron, niacin, thiamin, vitamins B6 and B12, folic acid, magnesium, and zinc. The amount of fat and number of calories varies, depending on what kind of meat or substitute. Both proteins and fat from the meat exchange are vital to normal health, and both have indirect effects on the level of blood sugar though the immediate effect on the blood sugar is minimal. The list is divided into three parts based on the amount of fat and calories.

## Lean Meat and Substitutes (3 grams of fat and 55 calories per serving)

| | | |
|---|---|---|
| Beef | USDA Select or Choice grades of lean beef, such as round, sirloin, and flank steak; tenderloin; roast (rib, chuck, rump); and chipped beef * | 1 oz |
| Pork | Lean pork, such as fresh ham; canned, cured, or boiled ham;* Canadian bacon,* tenderloin, center loin chop | 1 oz |
| Veal | All cuts are lean except for veal cutlets (ground or cubed); examples of lean veal are chops and roasts | 1 oz |
| Poultry | Chicken, turkey, Cornish hen (without skin) | 1 oz |
| Lamb | Roast, chop, leg | 1 oz |
| Fish | All fresh and frozen fish | 1 oz |
| | Crab, lobster, scallops, shrimp, clams (fresh or canned in water) | 2 oz |
| | Oysters | 6 medium |
| | Tuna† (canned in water) | 1/4 cup |
| | Herring† (uncreamed or smoked) | 1 oz |
| | Sardines (canned) | 2 medium |
| Wild | Game Venison, rabbit, squirrel | 1 oz |
| | Pheasant, duck, goose (without skin) | 1 oz |
| Cheese | Any cottage cheese† | 1/4 cup |
| | Grated parmesan | 2 tbsp |
| | Diet cheese* (with less than 55 calories per oz) | 1 oz |
| Other | 95% fat-free luncheon meat* | 1 1/2 oz |
| | Egg whites | 3 whites |

Egg substitutes with less than 55                    1/2 cup
calories per 1/2 cup

**Medium-Fat Meat and Substitutes (5 grams of fat and 75 calories per serving)**

Beef     Most beef products fall into this category;   1 oz
         examples are all ground beef, roast (rib,
         chuck, rump), steak (cubed, Porterhouse,
         T-bone), and meatloaf

Pork     Most pork products fall into this category;   1 oz
         examples are chops, loin roast, Boston
         butt, cutlets

Lamb     Most lamb products fall into this category;   1 oz
         examples are chops, leg, and roast

Veal     Cutlet (ground or cubed, unbreaded)           1 oz

Poultry  Chicken (with skin), domestic duck or         1 oz
         goose (well drained of fat), ground turkey

Fish     Tuna† (canned in oil and drained)             1/4 cup
         Salmon† (canned)

Cheese   Skim or part-skim milk cheeses, such as       1 oz
         Ricotta, mozzarella, and diet cheeses*
         (with 56–80 calories per oz)

Other    86% fat-free luncheon meats                   1 oz
         Egg (high in cholesterol, limit to            1
           3 per week)
         Egg substitutes with 56–80 calories per cup  1/4 cup
         Tofu (21/2 in. by 2 3/4 in. by 1 in.)         4 oz
         Liver, heart, kidney, sweetbreads (high in    1 oz
           cholesterol)

**High-Fat Meat and Substitutes (8 grams of fat and 100 calories per serving)**

Beef     Most USDA Prime cuts of beef,                 1 oz
           such as ribs, corned beef†

Pork     Spareribs, ground pork, pork                  1 oz
           sausages (patty or link)

| Lamb | Patties (ground lamb) | 1 oz |
| Fish | Any fried fish product (unbreaded) | 1 oz |
| Cheese | All regular cheeses, such as American,* blue,* cheddar,† Monterey jack,† Swiss | 1 oz |
| Other | Luncheon meat such as bologna, salami, pimento loaf | 1 oz |
| | Sausage,* such as Polish, Italian, smoked | 1 oz |
| | Knockwurst* | 1 oz |
| | Bratwurst† | |
| | Frankfurter* (turkey or chicken) | 1 frank |
| | Frankfurter* (beef, pork, or combination) (*Count as one high-fat meat plus one fat exchange.*) | 1 frank |
| | Peanut butter (contains unsaturated fat) | 1 tbsp |

*400 mg or more of sodium per exchange.
†400 mg or more of sodium if two or more exchanges are eaten.

---

### *Fat Exchange List*

Each serving in the fat list contains about 5 grams of fat and 45 calories. These foods contain mostly fat, but some items also contain protein. Fats provide essential fatty acids for healthy skin and development of body cells and a rich source of fat-soluble vitamins A, D, E, and K. Although vital to health, saturated fats have been linked to heart disease and cancer, and should be limited in the diet. Both proteins and fat from the fat exchange have indirect effects on the level of blood sugar, but the immediate effect on the blood sugar is minimal.

**Unsaturated Fats**

| | |
|---|---|
| Avocado | 1/8 medium |
| Margarine: stick or tub | 1 tsp |
| Margarine, lower fat† | 1 tbsp |
| Mayonnaise | 1 tsp |
| Mayonnaise, reduced calorie† | 1 tbsp |
| Nuts and seeds | 6 whole |
|    Almonds, dry roasted | 1 tbsp |
|    Cashews, dry roasted | |

| | |
|---|---|
| Pecans | 2 whole or 4 halves |
| Peanuts | 20 small or 10 large |
| Walnuts | 2 whole |
| Other nuts | 1 tbsp |
| Seeds, pine nuts, sunflower (without shells), pumpkin, and sesame seeds | 1 tbsp |
| Tahini paste | 2 tsp |
| Oil (corn, cottonseed, safflower, soybean, sunflower, olive, peanut) | 1 tsp |
| Olives* | 10 small or 8 large |
| Salad dressing, mayonnaise type* | 2 tsp |
| Salad dressing, mayonnaise type, reduced calorie | 1 tbsp |
| Salad dressing, reduced calorie* | 2 tbsp |
| Salad dressing (oil varieties)† | 1 tbsp |

(*Two tablespoons of low-calorie salad dressing is a free food—that is, any food or drink that contains fewer than 20 calories per serving.*)

**Saturated Fats**

| | |
|---|---|
| Butter, stick | 1 tsp |
| Butter, whipped | 1 tsp |
| Butter, reduced fat | 2 tsp |
| Bacon† | 1 slice |
| Chitterlings | 1/2 oz (2 tbsp) |
| Coconut, shredded | 2 tbsp |
| Coffee whitener, liquid | 2 tbsp |
| Coffee whitener, powder | 4 tsp |
| Cream (light, coffee, table) | 2 tbsp |
| Cream, half and half | 2 tbsp |
| Cream, sour | 2 tbsp |
| Cream, sour, reduced fat | 3 tbsp |
| Cream (heavy, whipping) | 1 tbsp |
| Cream cheese | 1 tbsp |
| Cream cheese, reduced fat | 2 tbsp |

Salt pork†                                                      1/4 oz
*400 mg or more of sodium per exchange.
†400 mg or more of sodium if two or more exchanges are eaten.

---

### Foods for Occasional Use and Fast Foods

Moderate amounts of some foods can be used in your meal plan, in spite of their sugar and fat content, as long as you maintain calorie and weight control. The following list includes average exchange values for some of these foods. Because they are concentrated sources of carbohydrate, and in some cases fat, you will notice that the portion sizes are very small.

| | |
|---|---|
| Angel food cake, 1/12 cake | 2 starch |
| Cake, no icing, 1/12 cake, or a 3 in. square | 2 starch, 2 fat |
| Cookies, 2 small (1 3/4 in. across) | 1 starch, 1 fat |
| Frozen fruit, 1/3 cup yogurt | 1 starch |
| Gingersnaps, 3 | 1 starch |
| Granola, 1/4 cup | 1 starch, 1 fat |
| Granola bars, 1 small | 1 starch, 1 fat |
| Ice cream, l/2 cup any flavor | 1 starch, 2 fat |
| Ice milk, 1/2 cup any flavor | 1 starch, 1 fat |
| Sherbet, 1/4 cup any flavor | 1 starch |
| Snack chips,* 1 oz all varieties | 1 starch, 2 fat |
| Vanilla wafers, 6 small | 1 starch |

*400 mg or more of sodium if two or more exchanges are eaten.

### Fast Foods

| | |
|---|---|
| Burritos with beef, 2* | 4 starch, 2 med-fat meats, 2 fats |
| Chicken nuggets, 6* | 1 starch, 2 med-fat meats, 1 fat |
| Chicken breast and wing, breaded and fried, 1 each* | 1 starch, 4 med-fat meats, 2 fats |
| Fish sandwich with tartar sauce, 1* | 3 starch, 1 med-fat meat, 3 fats |
| French fries, thin, 20–25* | 2 starch, 2 fats |
| Hamburger, regular, 1* | 2 starch, 2 med-fat meats |
| Hamburger, large, 1* | 2 starch, 3 med-fat meats, 1 fat |

| Hot dog with bun, 1* | 1 starch, 1 high-fat meat, 1 fat |
| Individual pan pizza, 1* | 5 starch, 3 med-fat meats, 3 fats |
| Self serve cone, | 1 medium 2 starch, 1 fat |
| Submarine sandwich, 1 sub (6 in.)* | 3 starch, 1 vegetable, 2 med-fat meats, 1 fat |
| Taco, hard shell, 1 (6 oz)* | 2 starch, 2 med-fat meats, 2 fats |
| Taco, soft shell, 1 (3 oz)* | 1 starch, 1 med-fat meat, 1 fat |

*400 mg or more of sodium per exchange.

---

### Combination Foods

Many foods do not fit into one exchange list and are categorized in the combination food list. This is a list of average values for some typical combination foods.

| Casseroles, homemade, 1 cup (8 oz) | 2 starch, 2 med-fat meat, 1 fat |
| Cheese pizza†, thin crust 1/4 of 15 oz or 1/4 of 10 in. 2 starch, | 1 med-fat meat, 1 fat |
| Chili with beans*† (commercial), 1 cup (8 oz) | 2 starch, 2 med-fat meat, 2 fat |
| Chow mein† (without noodles or rice), 2 cups (16 oz) | 1 starch, 2 vegetable, 2 lean meat |
| Macaroni and cheese,† 1 cup (8 oz) 2 starch, | 1 med-fat meat, 2 fat |
| Soup, 1 cup (8 oz) | 1 starch, 1 vegetable, 1 lean meat |
| Bean*† | 1 starch, 1 vegetable, 1 med-fat meat |
| Chunky, all varieties,† 10 3/4 oz can | 1 starch, 1 fat |
| Cream† (made with water), 1 cup (8 oz) | 1 starch |
| Vegetable† or broth-type,† 1 cup (8 oz) | 1 starch |
| Spaghetti and meatballs† (canned), 1 cup (8 oz) | 2 starch, 1 med-fat meat, 1 fat |

Sugar-free pudding, 1/2 cup
   (made with skim milk)          1 starch
*3 grams or more of fiber per exchange.
†400 mg or more of sodium per exchange.

---

### *Free Foods List*

A free food is any food or drink that contains fewer than 20 calories per serving. You can eat as much as you want of those items that have no serving size specified. You may eat two or three servings per day of those items that have a specific serving size.

Drinks
Bouillon or broth without fat
Bouillon, low sodium
Carbonated drinks, sugar-free
Carbonated water
Club soda
Cocoa powder, unsweetened (1 tbsp)
Coffee or tea
Drink mixes, sugar-free
Tonic water, sugar-free
Nonstick cooking spray
Fruit
Cranberries, unsweetened (1/2 cup)
Rhubarb, unsweetened (1/2 cup)
Vegetables (raw, 1 cup)
Cabbage
Celery
Chinese cabbage*
Cucumber
Green onion
Hot peppers
Mushrooms
Radishes
Zucchini*
Salad greens

Endive
Escarole
Lettuce
Romaine
Spinach
Sweet substitutes
Candy, hard, sugar-free
Gelatin, sugar-free
Gum, sugar-free
Jam or jelly, sugar-free (less than 20 cal per 2 tsp)
Pancake syrup, sugar-free (1–2 tbsp)
Sugar substitutes (saccharin, aspartame)
Whipped topping (2 tbsp)
Condiments
Catsup (1 tbsp)
Horseradish
Mustard
Pickles,† dill, unsweetened
Salad dressing, low calorie (2 tbsp)
Taco sauces (3 tbsp)
Vinegar

Seasonings can be very helpful in making food taste better. Be careful of how much sodium you use. Read the label, and choose those seasonings that do not contain sodium or salt.

Basil (fresh)
Celery seeds
Chili powder
Chives
Cinnamon
Curry
Dill
Flavoring extracts (vanilla, almond, walnut, peppermint, butter, lemon, and so forth)
Garlic
Garlic powder

Herbs
Hot pepper sauce
Lemon
Lemon juice
Lemon pepper
Lime
Lime juice
Mint
Onion powder
Oregano
Paprika
Pepper
Pimento
Spices
Soy sauce†
Soy sauce,† low sodium ("lite")
Wine, used in cooking (1/4 cup)
Worcestershire sauce

# Nineteen

## CALCULATING YOUR DAILY CALORIES AND BMI (BODY MASS INDEX)

HERE IS THE CALCULATION TABLE used to determine the proper number of calories you should have per day, along with the number of grams of protein, carbohydrates, and fats.

### Calculate Your Percentages

1 gram of protein = 4 calories
1 gram of carbohydrate = 4 calories
1 gram of fat = 9 calories

|  | You | Example (a forty-year-old) |
|---|---|---|
| Enter your weight here: | _____ | 210 |
| Multiply total by 10 | _____ | 2100 |
| Subtract 100 for every 10 years over 30 | _____ | -100 |
| total number of calories | _____ | 2000 |

The total you get is the amount of calories you need each day to stay the weight that you currently are. If you eat more, you will gain weight because it is more than your body needs. In order to lose weight, you must eat fewer calories than this, but no less than 1400 calories per day! Start with a small decrease in the number of calories that you eat.

Now, we must figure out the percentages (60 percent carbohy-drates, 30 percent protein, and 10 percent fat). In our example, the total calories we have decided on are 1600 (400 less than our body needs).

**Our Example**

If you eat four meals per day:

| | |
|---|---|
| Divide your total number of calories per day by 4 | 1600 / 4 = 400 calories per meal |

To calculate calories:

| | |
|---|---|
| Multiply the total number of calories per meal by .60 (60%) | 400 X .60 = 240 calories |
| Divide that total by 4 for the number of grams per meal | 240 / 4 = 60 grams |

For Protein:

| | |
|---|---|
| Multiply the total number of calories per meal by .30 | 400 X .30 = 120 |
| Divide that total by 4 for the number of grams per meal | 120 / 4 = 30 grams |

For Fat:

| | |
|---|---|
| Multiply the total number of calories per meal by .10 | 400 X .10 = 40 |
| Divide that total by 9 for the number of grams per meal | 40 / 9 = approx. 5 grams |

Each of these calculations results in the number of calories per meal for each nutrient, and the number of grams per nutrient. On almost all food products you buy, the "Nutrition Facts" label lists each nutrient, along with the number of grams per serving.

# *Appendix A*

# ADDITIONAL EXERCISES

***Lateral Shoulder Raises*** are for toning and strengthening your shoulders. Using lightweight dumbbells, stand with your feet shoulder length apart. Keeping your back straight lift the dumbbells slowly until arms are parallel to the floor. Keeping tension on the shoulders, lower the dumbbells slowly until arms are resting at your side. Repeat for 10 repetitions. Try to do 3 sets of 10's.

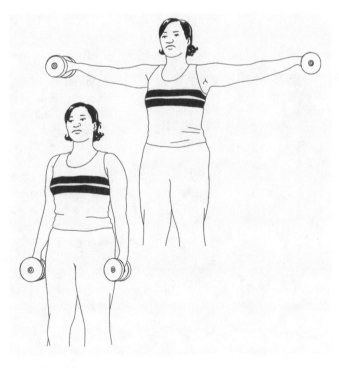

***Standing Lunges*** are for toning and tightening your thighs. Standing with your back straight, hold the dumbbells firmly in your hands and make sure your feet are shoulder width apart. Take a small step forward, being careful not to extend your knee over your foot (injury can result if your knee is extended too far or you take a step that is too far). You should feel the tension in the top of your leg, which is your thigh muscle. Then step back to your original position. Reverse and do the other leg. Try to build up to 10 on each leg. These can be difficult in the beginning. Practice them slowly and be patient.

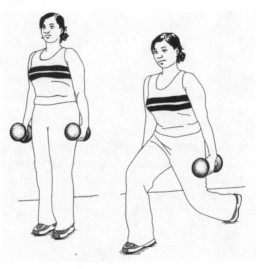

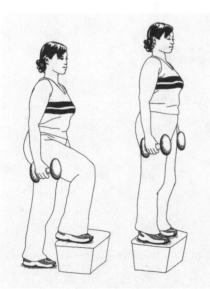

***Step-ups*** are for toning and tightening your thigh muscles. These are a little less difficult than standing lunges, but once you get going you'll be able to do both exercises on the same day of your workout. Find a box that is sturdy or simply use your porch steps or staircase. Make sure to keep your back straight while stepping up. Once you step up stand still for a moment before stepping down. Alternate using the other leg. Try to do 10 on each leg.

***Sitting Dumbbell Raises.*** This exercise can build tone in your shoulders. Sit with
your back straight and hold the dumbbells firmly in your hands with your elbows
slightly bent. Lift slowly until your arms are extended above your head. Slowly return
to the starting position and keeping tension in the shoulder area. Repeat for 10 repetitions. Do 3 sets.

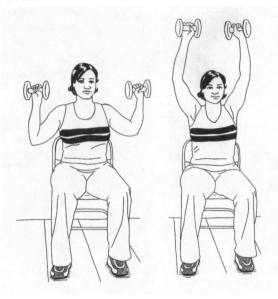

***Push-ups*** are for strengthening
your chest muscles. Women tend
to have less strength in their
chests but by doing exercises for
your upper body posture will
improve. With your knees firmly
on the floor and your arms
placed slightly wider than your
shoulders, bend down and touch
your chest to the floor. Return to
the starting position. Concentrate
on keeping your back straight to
avoid injury. Do 3 sets of 10 repetitions.

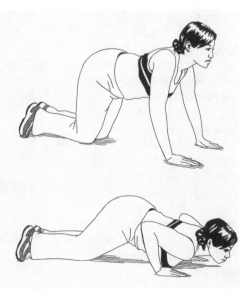

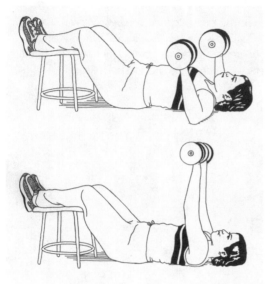

***Dumbbell Presses***. This exercise is for your chest and shoulders. Lying on the floor with your legs supported on a bench, firmly hold the dumbbells over your elbows. The elbows resting on the floor will aid in support of the weight. Lift the dumbbells slowly until your arms are extended upward without locking your elbows. Return to the starting position and repeat 10 times. Do 3 sets.

***Alternating Dumbbell Curls.*** These exercises will build up your biceps and upper arms. Rest the dumbbells at your side with palms facing toward your thighs. Rotate at the elbow joint and bring the weight up to your chest. Do these slowly to keep tension on the muscle. Lower the dumbbell to the starting position keeping tension on the muscle (Remember that constant tension is what causes the muscle to become stronger). Alternate and do the same movement for the other arm. Do 3 sets and 10 repetitions on each arm.

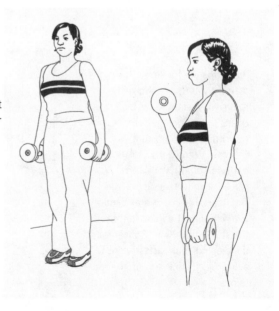

**Bent Over Rows** for your back. Bend over slightly and support your weight by placing a hand firmly on the seat of a chair. Keep your back straight and allow the dumbbell to hang down almost touching the chair. Lift the weight slowly until the dumbbell touches the outside of your chest. Make sure to keep your back straight to avoid injury. You can do 10 and then alternate and do 10 repetitions using the other arm. Do 3 sets.

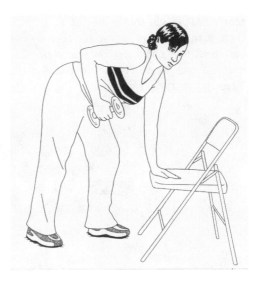

**Standing Leg Presses** against the wall. These will build up your thighs and place less stress on your back. Stand with your back against a wall, making sure your feet are positioned a foot away from the wall. Slide down the wall until your thighs are parallel to the floor. Make sure that your knees are not extended beyond your feet. Keeping the tension on your thighs slide back up the wall to the starting position. Repeat 10 times. Do 3 sets.

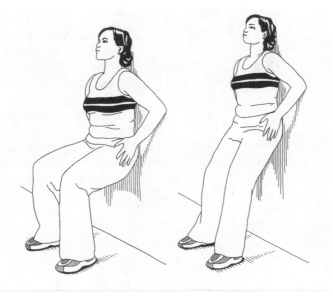

**Modified Push-ups** against the wall. Push-ups will tone, tighten and lift your chest. Place your palms against the wall and extend your arms straight by walking backwards. In this position allow your elbows to bend while you lower your chest until it touches the wall. Lift off the wall slowly to the starting position. Repeat for 10 repetitions. Do 3 sets.

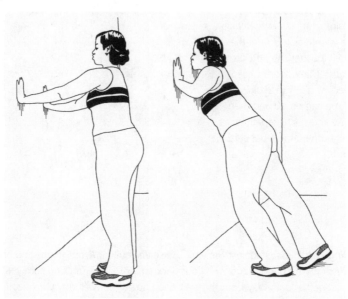

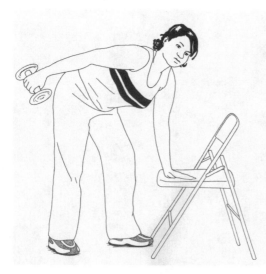

**Dumbbell Kick-Backs** are for the triceps. Bend over a chair keeping your back straight, and allow the dumbbell to hang down close to the chair. Rotating only at the elbow, extend the dumbbell backwards until your elbow is almost locked. Keep the tension on the back of your arm. Do 10 repetitions on each arm for 3 sets.

## *Appendix B*

# Planners, Logs, and List

Meal Planner

Daily Food Diary

Aerobic Activity Log

Strength Training Log

Healthy Grocery List

## MEAL PLANNER

MEAL PLAN FOR THE WEEK OF:

| | Sunday 11/16 | Monday 11/17 | Tuesday 11/18 | Wednesday 11/19 | Thursday 11/20 | Friday 11/21 | Saturday 11/22 |
|---|---|---|---|---|---|---|---|
| | Breakfast | Breakfast | Breakfast | Breakfast | Breakfast | Breakfast | Breakfast |
| | Calories:<br>Fat grams: | Calories:<br>Fat grams: | Calories:<br>Fat grams: | Calories:<br>Fat grams: | Calories:<br>Fat grams: | Calories:<br>Fat grams: | Calories:<br>Fat grams: |
| | Lunch | Lunch | Lunch | Lunch | Lunch | Lunch | Lunch |
| | Calories:<br>Fat grams: | Calories:<br>Fat grams: | Calories:<br>Fat grams: | Calories:<br>Fat grams: | Calories:<br>Fat grams: | Calories:<br>Fat grams: | Calories:<br>Fat grams: |
| | Dinner | Dinner | Dinner | Dinner | Dinner | Dinner | Dinner |
| | Calories:<br>Fat grams: | Calories:<br>Fat grams: | Calories:<br>Fat grams: | Calories:<br>Fat grams: | Calories:<br>Fat grams: | Calories:<br>Fat grams: | Calories:<br>Fat grams: |
| | Snack | Snack | Snack | Snack | Snack | Snack | Snack |
| | Calories:<br>Fat grams: | Calories:<br>Fat grams: | Calories:<br>Fat grams: | Calories:<br>Fat grams: | Calories:<br>Fat grams: | Calories:<br>Fat grams: | Calories:<br>Fat grams: |
| | Calories:<br>Fat grams:<br>% calories<br>from fat | Calories:<br>Fat grams:<br>% calories<br>from fat | Calories:<br>Fat grams:<br>% calories<br>from fat | Calories:<br>Fat grams:<br>% calories<br>from fat | Calories:<br>Fat grams:<br>% calories<br>from fat | Calories:<br>Fat grams:<br>% calories<br>from fat | Calories:<br>Fat grams:<br>% calories<br>from fat |

**Weekly Total**

Calories: 0
Fat grams: 0
% calories from fat 0.0%

# DAILY FOOD DIARY

| NAME: | Maximum Daily Calories: |
| DATE: | Maximum Daily Fat Grams: |

| | Fod Eaten | Amount | Fat Grams | Calories | Comment |
|---|---|---|---|---|---|
| **Breakfast** | Granola | 1/2 cup | 2 | 160 | |
| | | | | | |
| | | | | | |
| | | | | | |
| | | | | | |
| | | | | | |
| **Snack** | Apple | 1 small | 0 | 60 | |
| | | | | | |
| **Lunch** | Sandwich | | 5 | 450 | |
| | | | | | |
| | | | | | |
| | | | | | |
| | | | | | |
| | | | | | |
| **Snack** | | | | | |
| | | | | | |
| **Dinner** | | | | | |
| | | | | | |
| | | | | | |
| | | | | | |
| | | | | | |
| | | | | | |
| **Snack** | | | | | |
| | | | | | |
| | | | | | |
| **Water** | ( )( )( )( )( )( )( )( ) | | | | |

|  | **Total** | 7 | 670 |
|---|---|---|---|

Percent fat consumed of total calories:   9%

Comments

_____

_____

_____

_____

_____

# AEROBIC ACTIVITY LOG

NAME: JANE
AGE: 32
START DATE: 6/6/01

| | Beats per minute | Beats per 10 seconds |
|---|---|---|
| 55% of your max. heart rate | 103 | 17 |
| 65% of your max. heart rate | 122 | 20 |
| 90% of your max. heart rate | 169 | 28 |

**Activity**

| | | 6/6 | 6/7 | 6/8 | 6/9 | 6/10 | 6/11 | 6/12 | 6/13 | 6/14 | 6/15 | 6/16 | 6/17 | 6/18 | 6/19 | 6/20 | 6/21 | 6/22 | 6/23 | 6/24 | 6/25 | 6/26 |
|---|---|---|---|---|---|---|---|---|---|---|---|---|---|---|---|---|---|---|---|---|---|---|
| Walking | minutes | 30 | | | | | | | | | | | | | | | | | | | | |
| | avg. heart rate | 120 | | | | | | | | | | | | | | | | | | | | |
| | minutes | | | | | | | | | | | | | | | | | | | | | |
| | minutes | | | | | | | | | | | | | | | | | | | | | |
| | avg. heart rate | | | | | | | | | | | | | | | | | | | | | |
| | minutes | | | | | | | | | | | | | | | | | | | | | |
| | minutes | | | | | | | | | | | | | | | | | | | | | |
| | avg. heart rate | | | | | | | | | | | | | | | | | | | | | |
| | minutes | | | | | | | | | | | | | | | | | | | | | |
| | minutes | | | | | | | | | | | | | | | | | | | | | |
| | avg. heart rate | | | | | | | | | | | | | | | | | | | | | |
| | minutes | | | | | | | | | | | | | | | | | | | | | |
| | minutes | | | | | | | | | | | | | | | | | | | | | |
| | avg. heart rate | | | | | | | | | | | | | | | | | | | | | |
| | minutes | | | | | | | | | | | | | | | | | | | | | |
| | minutes | | | | | | | | | | | | | | | | | | | | | |
| | avg. heart rate | | | | | | | | | | | | | | | | | | | | | |
| | minutes | | | | | | | | | | | | | | | | | | | | | |
| | minutes | | | | | | | | | | | | | | | | | | | | | |
| | avg. heart rate | | | | | | | | | | | | | | | | | | | | | |
| | minutes | | | | | | | | | | | | | | | | | | | | | |
| | minutes | | | | | | | | | | | | | | | | | | | | | |
| | avg. heart rate | | | | | | | | | | | | | | | | | | | | | |
| | minutes | | | | | | | | | | | | | | | | | | | | | |

## STRENGTH TRAINING LOG EXAMPLE

NAME:

START DATE:   6/6/01

| Exercise | | 6/6 | 6/7 | 6/8 | 6/9 | 6/10 | 6/11 | 6/12 | 6/13 | 6/14 | 6/15 | 6/16 | 6/17 | 6/18 | 6/19 | 6/20 | 6/21 | 6/22 | 6/23 | 6/24 | 6/25 | 6/26 |
|---|---|---|---|---|---|---|---|---|---|---|---|---|---|---|---|---|---|---|---|---|---|---|
| | lbs. | | | | | | | | | | | | | | | | | | | | | |
| | reps. | | | | | | | | | | | | | | | | | | | | | |
| | lbs. | | | | | | | | | | | | | | | | | | | | | |
| | reps. | | | | | | | | | | | | | | | | | | | | | |
| | lbs. | | | | | | | | | | | | | | | | | | | | | |
| | reps. | | | | | | | | | | | | | | | | | | | | | |
| | lbs. | | | | | | | | | | | | | | | | | | | | | |
| | reps. | | | | | | | | | | | | | | | | | | | | | |
| | lbs. | | | | | | | | | | | | | | | | | | | | | |
| | reps. | | | | | | | | | | | | | | | | | | | | | |
| | lbs. | | | | | | | | | | | | | | | | | | | | | |
| | reps. | | | | | | | | | | | | | | | | | | | | | |
| | lbs. | | | | | | | | | | | | | | | | | | | | | |
| | reps. | | | | | | | | | | | | | | | | | | | | | |
| | lbs. | | | | | | | | | | | | | | | | | | | | | |
| | reps. | | | | | | | | | | | | | | | | | | | | | |
| | lbs. | | | | | | | | | | | | | | | | | | | | | |
| | reps. | | | | | | | | | | | | | | | | | | | | | |
| | lbs. | | | | | | | | | | | | | | | | | | | | | |
| | reps. | | | | | | | | | | | | | | | | | | | | | |
| | lbs. | | | | | | | | | | | | | | | | | | | | | |
| | reps. | | | | | | | | | | | | | | | | | | | | | |

# HEALTHY GROCERY LIST

DATE: _____

## Dairy

- ❑ _____ Eggs
- ❑ _____ Milk (skim)
- ❑ _____ Spray Butter
- ❑ _____ Sour Cream (fat free)
- ❑ _____ Yogurt
- ❑ _____ Cottage Cheese
- ❑ _____ Cream Cheese (fat free)
- ❑ _____ Parmesan Cheese
- ❑ _____ Other Cheese (fat free)
- ❑ _____ _____

## Meat, Fish, & Poultry

- ❑ _____ Turkey Bacon
- ❑ _____ Turkey Sausage
- ❑ _____ Deli Meat
- ❑ _____ Hot Dogs (fat free)
- ❑ _____ Chicken (Breast)
- ❑ _____ Turkey
- ❑ _____ Beef (choice cuts)
- ❑ _____ Pork (loin or white)
- ❑ _____ Fish
- ❑ _____ Shellfish
- ❑ _____ _____

## Fruit

- ❑ _____ Apples
- ❑ _____ Bananas
- ❑ _____ Berries
- ❑ _____ Grapefruit
- ❑ _____ Grapes
- ❑ _____ Lemons
- ❑ _____ Limes
- ❑ _____ Melon
- ❑ _____ Oranges
- ❑ _____ Pears
- ❑ _____ Vegetable
- ❑ _____ Broccoli
- ❑ _____ Cabbage
- ❑ _____ Carrots
- ❑ _____ Cauliflower
- ❑ _____ Celery
- ❑ _____ Cucumbers
- ❑ _____ Garlic

- ❑ _____ Lettuce
- ❑ _____ Mushrooms
- ❑ _____ Onions
- ❑ _____ Peppers
- ❑ _____ Potatoes
- ❑ _____ Radishes Spinach
- ❑ _____ Tomatoes
- ❑ _____ _____

## Breads

- ❑ _____ Bagels (small)
- ❑ _____ Bread (whole wheat)
- ❑ _____ English Muffins
- ❑ _____ _____

## Dry Goods

- ❑ _____ Cereal (low sugar)
- ❑ _____ Oatmeal
- ❑ _____ Crackers (fat free)
- ❑ _____ Pasta/Noodles
- ❑ _____ Beans/Lentils/Peas Rice
- ❑ _____ Bread Crumbs
- ❑ _____ Flour
- ❑ _____ Sugar (Equal)
- ❑ _____ Cake Mix (Angel Food)
- ❑ _____ Pancake Mix
- ❑ _____ Gelatin
- ❑ _____ Potato Chips (fat free)
- ❑ _____ Tortilla Chips (fat free)
- ❑ _____ _____

## Canned Goods

- ❑ _____ Applesauce
- ❑ _____ Fruit
- ❑ _____ Mushrooms
- ❑ _____ Soup (Healthy Choice)
- ❑ _____ Spaghetti Sauce
- ❑ _____ Stewed Tomatoes
- ❑ _____ Tomato Paste
- ❑ _____ Tomato Sauce
- ❑ _____ Tuna
- ❑ _____ Vegetables
- ❑ _____ _____

## Frozen Foods

- ❑ _____ Frozen Yogurt (fat free)
- ❑ _____ Potatoes
- ❑ _____ Vegetables (low salt)
- ❑ _____ Frozen Dinners
- ❑ _____ Frozen Waffles
- ❑ _____ _____

## Baking Goods

- ❑ _____ Baking Soda
- ❑ _____ Baking Powder
- ❑ _____ Corn Starch
- ❑ _____ Salt
- ❑ _____ Pepper
- ❑ _____ Nuts
- ❑ _____ Raisins
- ❑ _____ Vanilla
- ❑ _____ Dried Herbs
- ❑ _____ Spices
- ❑ _____ _____

## Condiments

- ❑ _____ Olive Oil
- ❑ _____ Vinegar
- ❑ _____ Ketchup
- ❑ _____ Mayonnaise (fat free)
- ❑ _____ Mustard
- ❑ _____ Olives
- ❑ _____ Pickles
- ❑ _____ Relish
- ❑ _____ Salsa
- ❑ _____ Salad Dressing (fat free)
- ❑ _____ Soy Sauce (low sodium)
- ❑ _____ Soy Sauce (low sodium)
- ❑ _____ Honey
- ❑ _____ Jelly/Jam
- ❑ _____ Syrup (sugar free)
- ❑ _____ _____

## Beverages

- ❑ _____ Coffee
- ❑ _____ Tea
- ❑ _____ Fruit Juice
- ❑ _____ Soft Drinks (diet)
- ❑ _____ Mineral Water
- ❑ _____ Wine
- ❑ _____ _____

## Paper products

- ❑ _____ Facial Tissue
- ❑ _____ Toilet Tissue
- ❑ _____ Napkins
- ❑ _____ Paper Towels
- ❑ _____ Aluminum Foil
- ❑ _____ Plastic Wrap
- ❑ _____ Lunch Bags
- ❑ _____ Sandwich Bags
- ❑ _____ Garbage Bags
- ❑ _____ _____

## Laundry

- ❑ _____ Bleach
- ❑ _____ Detergent
- ❑ _____ Fabric Softener
- ❑ _____ Stain Remover
- ❑ _____ _____

## Kitchen

- ❑ _____ All Purpose Cleaner
- ❑ _____ Dish Detergent
- ❑ _____ Dishwasher Soap
- ❑ _____ Floor Cleaner
- ❑ _____ Furniture Polish
- ❑ _____ Glass Cleaner
- ❑ _____ Steel Wool Pads
- ❑ _____ _____

## Bathroom

- ❑ _____ Bath Soap
- ❑ _____ Deodorant
- ❑ _____ Lotion
- ❑ _____ Razors
- ❑ _____ Shaving Cream
- ❑ _____ Shampoo
- ❑ _____ Toothpaste
- ❑ _____ _____

## Miscellaneous

Bandages          Batteries
Candles           Light Bulbs
Paper Plates      Pet Food
Stamps            Vitamins
- ❑ _____ _____

# *Appendix C*

# RECIPES FOR HEALTHY LIVING

## BREAKFAST RECIPES

B REAKFAST IS THE MOST IMPORTANT MEAL of the day. It provides you with the fuel you need to get your body, and your brain, started. Too often, people skip breakfast, thinking that they will just grab a bite to eat at lunch. There is a rebound effect from not eating something at breakfast. Your blood sugar drops, and your concentration levels suffer. Faced with an energy deficit, your body begins to store fat instead of burn it for energy.

The foods you choose for breakfast are not as important as the nutrients they supply.

Many lowfat cereals can be eaten with skim milk. If you want something from the bread, cereal, rice and pasta group from the Food Guide Pyramid, select something that is low in saturated fat. Fresh fruits are a good choice. Jams, jellies, and preserves are high in carbohydrates and do not give you the same nutrients that fresh fruit provides.

Choices from the meat, poultry, fish, dried beans, eggs and nuts group for breakfast are limited. These foods are generally high in calories and fat.

### Tropical Fruit Cup

2 bananas, peeled and sliced
1/4 lb grapefruit pieces
1/2 lb unsweetened pineapple chunks
1/2 lb guava halves

Combine all ingredients in a bowl. Cover and chill 30 minutes.

Serves 1

Nutritive Information per Serving
Calories:                148
Protein (g):               2
Fat (g):                   1
Carbohydrates (g):        37

### Grilled Pineapple Slices

2 tbsp brown sugar
6 fresh pineapple slices, 1/2 in. thick each

Prepare grill.

Sprinkle brown sugar onto pineapple slices and place on grill over medium heat.

Cook about 10 minutes, turning slices occasionally, until browned on both sides.

Serves 4

Nutritive Information per Serving
Calories:                 71
Protein (g):               1
Fat (g):                   0
Carbohydrates (g):        19

### Fat-Free Pumpkin Muffins

nonstick cooking spray
1 cup canned cooked pumpkin

1 cup bran cereal shreds, crushed
3/4 cup skim milk
1/3 cup light or dark corn syrup
2 egg whites, slightly beaten
1 1/4 cups all-purpose flour
1/3 cup sugar
2 tsp baking powder
1/2 tsp salt
1/2 cup raisins

Preheat oven to 400°F. Spray twelve 2 1/2 in. muffin cups with cooking spray.

Combine pumpkin and next four ingredients in a bowl. Combine remaining ingredients in another bowl. Add pumpkin mixture and stir until well blended. Spoon into prepared muffin cups. Bake 20 minutes, or until toothpick inserted in center comes out clean. Cool in pan 5 minutes. Remove and cool on wire rack.

Serves 12

Nutritive Information per Serving
Calories:                138
Protein (g):               3
Fat (g):                   3
Carbohydrates (g):        33

### Creamy Tropical Shake

2 oranges, peeled and quartered
2 bananas, peeled
2 cups green or red seedless grapes
12 ice cubes, crushed
2 tsp honey
1/2 cup green or red seedless grapes

Place first three ingredients in a blender or food processor and process until smooth. Add ice cubes and honey, and blend. Pour into glasses. Sprinkle with extra grapes as a garnish if desired.

Serves 4

Nutritive Information per Serving
Calories:        193
Protein (g):      2
Fat (g):        1
Carbohydrates (g):  49

### Microwave Fruity Oatmeal

1 1/3 cups oatmeal, uncooked
2 2/3 cups water
2 packets equal
1 tsp cinnamon
1 apple, chopped
1 tbsp plus 1 tsp currants or raisins
1 tbsp plus 1 tsp chopped walnuts
1 cup skim milk

Combine all ingredients, except milk, in a microwave-safe bowl. Microwave on high 2 minutes. Serve with milk.

Serves 1

Nutritive Information per Serving
Calories:        181
Protein (g):      7
Fat (g):        3
Carbohydrates (g):  32

### New Zealand French Toast

2 egg whites
1/3 cup nonfat milk
1 tsp cinnamon
1 slice whole grain bread
1 slice nonfat cheese
1 kiwifruit, sliced

Heat a nonstick skillet over medium heat. Beat egg whites and milk in a square or rectangular container, then stir in cinnamon. Soak bread in egg-white mixture, transfer to skillet and brown on both sides. Top with cheese and cook until cheese is slightly melted. Add kiwi on top or on the side.

Serves 1

Nutritive Information per Serving
Calories:              233
Protein (g):            23
Fat (g):                 1
Carbohydrates (g):      33

### Egg-White Pancakes

6 jumbo egg whites
1 rounded tsp pancake mix
1 packet instant oatmeal or grits
nonstick cooking oil

Put the egg whites, pancake mix, and packet of oatmeal or grits in a blender. Blend until smooth. Pour mixture into a heated Teflon pan sprayed with nonstick cooking oil. Cook on medium heat for 11 minutes. Flip it over and cook until it is done.

Serves 1

Nutritive Information per Serving
Calories:              240
Protein (g):            26
Fat (g):                 1
Carbohydrates (g):      37

## LUNCH RECIPES

### Turkey Breast Sandwich

4.4 oz turkey breast fillet
1/2 tsp pepper

nonstick cooking spray
8 slices whole wheat bread
1/2 cup barbecue sauce
1/2 cup sliced sweet pickles
4 romaine lettuce leaves
1 tomato, sliced

Season turkey with pepper. Place turkey fillets between two sheets of wax paper and pound lightly with a mallet or other heavy flat object until very thin. Coat a heavy nonstick skillet with nonstick cooking spray and place over medium-high heat. Sauté turkey 2–3 minutes per side, until lightly browned and cooked throughout.

Nutritive Information per Serving
Calories:              362
Protein (g):            35
Fat (g):                 4
Carbohydrates (g):      42

Serves 4

### Curried Waldorf Salad

2 Red Delicious apples, cored and diced
1 Granny Smith apple, cored and diced
3/4 cup celery, sliced
1/3 cup raisins
1 tbsp walnuts, chopped
1 1/2 tsp curry powder
1/8 tsp pepper, or to taste
1/3 cup vanilla yogurt

Combine first five ingredients in a bowl and toss. Combine curry powder with the remaining ingredients. Add to apple mixture, tossing gently to coat.

Serves 4

Nutritive Information per Serving
Calories:              143

Protein (g):         2
Fat (g):             2
Carbohydrates (g):   33

### Creamy Cucumber Salad

1 lb European or garden salad
1 large green bell pepper, seeded and cut into thin strips
1 cup cherry tomatoes
1/2 cup fat-free creamy cucumber dressing
1 cup cool herb croutons

Combine all ingredients in a salad bowl and toss.

Serves 4

Nutritive Information per Serving
Calories:            127
Protein (g):         4
Fat (g):             2
Carbohydrates (g):   24

### Mixed Salad with Thousand Island Dressing

1/2 lb garden salad
2 cups spinach leaves, washed and torn into pieces, tough stems
    discarded
1/2 cup mushrooms, sliced
1 cup cherry tomatoes
1/2 green bell pepper, seeded and cut into 1 inch pieces
1/4 cup fat-free Thousand Island dressing
1 cup cool herb croutons

Combine first five ingredients in a salad bowl. Add dressing and pepper to taste and toss. Serve with croutons.

Serves 4

Nutritive Information per Serving
Calories:            121

Protein (g):              6
Fat (g):                  3
Carbohydrates (g):       21


### *Chicken Salad*

2 cups cooked rice, cooled
2 cups cantaloupe, cubed
1 1/2 cups cooked chicken breast, cubed
1/4 cup fresh mint, finely chopped
1/4 cup fresh parsley, finely chopped
1 clove garlic, finely chopped
1/2 lb plain nonfat yogurt
4 lettuce leaves

Mix first three ingredients in a bowl. Combine next four ingredients in another bowl. Gently stir yogurt mixture into rice mixture until well combined. Cover and refrigerate at least 2 hours, until chilled. Serve lettuce on individual plates topped with chicken salad.

Serves 4

Nutritive Information per Serving
Calories:               278
Protein (g):             23
Fat (g):                  3
Carbohydrates (g):       39


### *Mom's Potato Salad*

2 1/2 lb small new potatoes
1 large egg, hard-cooked, peeled, and chopped
3 tbsp fat-free mayonnaise
3 tbsp nonfat sour cream
1/4 cup dill relish
1 tbsp scallions, finely chopped

2 tbsp prepared mustard
1 tsp dried tarragon

Place potatoes in a steamer basket over boiling water. Cover pan
and steam about 20 minutes, or until just tender. Drain potatoes
and rinse under cold running water to cool. Combine remaining
ingredients with salt and pepper to taste in a bowl. Peel potatoes
and cut into 1/2 in. dice, and gently toss with egg mixture. Serve
potato salad chilled or at room temperature.

Serves 8

Nutritive Information per Serving
Calories:                  160
Protein (g):                 4
Fat (g):                     1
Carbohydrates (g):          34


### Turkey Sandwich with Cranberry-Orange Relish
1/4 cup plus 2 tbsp purchased cranberry orange relish, or
    homemade
1/4 cup celery, finely chopped
2 tbsp plus 2 tsp fat-free mayonnaise
8 slices cinnamon raisin bread, toasted
12 slices cooked turkey breast

Combine relish and celery in a bowl. Stir well and set aside. Spread
a portion of mayonnaise over each bread slice. Divide turkey
between half the bread slices. Spoon cranberry mixture over turkey
and top with remaining bread.

Serves 4

Nutritive Information per Serving
Calories:                  280
Protein (g):                18
Fat (g):                     4
Carbohydrates (g):          44

### *Microwave Miso Soup*

1 shiitake or portabello mushroom, stemmed and thinly sliced
4 cups fish stock or clam juice (chicken broth can be substituted
    for this)
1/4 cup miso paste
1/4 lb tofu, cut into 1/2 in. cubes
2 scallions, trimmed and cut into 2 in. lengths

Combine first two ingredients in a microwave-safe bowl. Cover
and microwave 5 minutes on high, or until mushroom is soft. Stir
in miso paste and tofu. Cover and microwave 2 minutes on high,
or until hot. Serve sprinkled with scallions.

Serves 4

Nutritive Information per Serving
Calories:                 106
Protein (g):               10
Fat (g):                    4
Carbohydrates (g):          8

### *Slow Cooker Cauliflower Soup*

1 lb cauliflower florets
1 3/4 lb canned diced tomatoes, undrained
14 oz vegetable or beef stock
1 onion, chopped
1/2 tsp garlic powder
2 tsp curry powder
1/8 tsp ground cumin

Combine first five ingredients in an electric slow cooker on low
heat. Cover and cook about 7 hours, or until cauliflower is tender.
Increase heat to high. Stir in remaining ingredients and salt and
pepper to taste. Cover and cook another 30 minutes. Serve hot or
cold.

Serves 4

Nutritive Information per Serving
Calories:                    90
Protein (g):                  5
Fat (g):                      1
Carbohydrates (g):           18


### Slow Cooker Brown Rice and Mushroom Soup

3/4 cup long grain brown rice
1/2 lb mushrooms, finely chopped
1 onion, finely chopped
1 celery stalk, finely chopped
1 tsp ground mustard
1 tsp fresh ground pepper
1/2 tsp salt
1/4 tsp ground coriander
1/8 tsp ground cardamom
1/8 tsp ground cinnamon
1/8 tsp ground cloves
1 quart plus 2 cups vegetable or chicken stock
1/3 cup fresh cilantro, chopped
1/2 cup nonfat plain yogurt or sour cream
3 tbsp scallions, finely chopped

Combine first twelve ingredients in slow cooker. Cover and cook on low 5–6 hours, or until rice is tender. Stir in cilantro. Serve topped with a dollop of yogurt and sprinkled with scallions.

Serves 8

Nutritive Information per Serving
Calories:                   100
Protein (g):                  4
Fat (g):                      1
Carbohydrates (g):           20

### *Cold Tomato Soup*

1 lb fresh or canned ripe tomatoes
3/4 medium green pepper, seeded and cut into pieces
1 1/4 small cucumbers, peeled, seeded, and cut into small pieces
2 tbsp plus 2 tsp red wine vinegar
1/8 tsp tarragon
1/8 tsp sugar
1 clove garlic, chopped
2/3 cup tomato juice
1/3 cup seasoned croutons

Place first eight ingredients and salt to taste in the bowl of a food processor or blender, in several steps if necessary. Blend until no large pieces remain. Strain, pressing with the back of a wooden spoon to extract as much liquid as possible. Correct the seasoning, adding more salt and vinegar if desired. Chill very well, preferably overnight. Serve with croutons.

Serves 4

Nutritive Information per Serving
Calories:            60
Protein (g):          3
Fat (g):              1
Carbohydrates (g):   13

### *Roasted Vegetable Soup*

8 tomatoes, cut in half
1 tbsp sugar
2 red onions, sliced
2 zucchini, sliced
2 yellow squash, sliced
3 red bell peppers, seeded and sliced
2 cloves garlic, chopped
2 tbsp rosemary, chopped
1 lemon, juiced

Preheat oven to 425°F. Arrange tomatoes cut side up in the bottom of an oiled nonreactive baking pan. Sprinkle with sugar. Combine remaining vegetables, garlic, and rosemary in another oiled baking pan. Season with salt and pepper to taste. Place both pans in oven and roast 25–30 minutes, stirring squash mixture every 8–10 minutes until vegetables are tender. Working in batches if necessary, combine tomatoes, lemon juice, and all but 1 cup of the vegetables in a food processor or blender. Process until smooth. Chop remaining vegetables and serve soup with chopped vegetables sprinkled on top.

Serves 6

Nutritive Information per Serving
Calories: 112
Protein (g): 5
Fat (g): 1
Carbohydrates (g): 28

### South-of-the-Border Bean Salad

16 oz whole green beans, drained
15 oz garbanzo beans, drained
15 oz kidney beans, drained
12 oz whole kernel corn with sweet peppers, drained
1 medium onion, chopped
1/2 cup fat-free French dressing (or any other fat-free salad dressing)
1/2 cup fat-free cheddar cheese, shredded
6 large lettuce leaves

Toss beans, corn, and onion with dressing in a large bowl. Refrigerate at least one hour or overnight. Before serving, toss with cheese and spoon onto lettuce leaves, either in salad bowls or on plates.

Serves 6

Nutritive Information per Serving
Calories:              252
Protein (g):            14
Fat (g):                 2
Carbohydrates (g):      45

### *Zesty Texas Chili*

1/2 cup chopped white onion
1 lb extremely lean ground beef or 1 lb extra-firm lowfat tofu,
    chopped
30 oz chili beans
16 oz crushed tomatoes
4 celery stalks, chopped
natural chili seasoning to taste
1 tsp dried or 2 tsp fresh cilantro
1 tsp balsamic vinegar
1/2 cup grated soy cheese, divided
Fresh parsley

In a large nonstick skillet, brown onion with ground beef or tofu over medium-high heat. Reduce heat to low, add next six ingredients and simmer until celery is soft. Transfer to four bowls; garnish each with cheese and parsley sprigs.

Serves 4

Nutritive Information per Serving (Beef)
Calories:              478
Protein (g):            50
Fat (g):                10
Carbohydrates (g):      47

Nutritive Information per Serving (Tofu)
Calories:              364
Protein (g):            27
Fat (g)                  8
Carbohydrates (g):      46

## Caesar Salad

1 egg (optional)
1 head romaine lettuce
3 tbsp olive oil
1 tbsp red wine vinegar
1 tbsp lemon juice
1/2–1 tsp Worcestershire sauce
1/2–3/4 tsp black pepper
1/4 tsp salt
1/4 cup parmesan cheese, grated

Coddle egg; set aside. Wash, then tear romaine into bite size pieces. Place in large bowl.

Sprinkle olive oil on romaine; toss. Sprinkle vinegar, lemon juice, Worcestershire sauce, pepper and salt on romaine; toss. Sprinkle with parmesan cheese and egg; toss. Toss in croutons; serve immediately.

Serves 4

Nutritive Information per Serving
Calories: 165
Protein (g): 5
Fat (g): 14
Carbohydrates (g): 5

## Chicken Alphabet Soup

1/2 chicken, cut into pieces
1 pkg vegetable soup mix with mushrooms
3–5 carrots, peeled and sliced
2–4 celery stalks, sliced
1/8–1/4 onion, finely chopped
6 cups water
salt and pepper, to taste
1/2 cup alphabet noodles

Place all ingredients, except alphabet noodles, in a large saucepan and bring the ingredients to a boil. Simmer over medium-low heat until dried vegetables are tender and chicken is cooked through (about 45 minutes to over 1 hour). Remove chicken from saucepan; allow to cool slightly; set aside. Remove any fat that may have floated to the top of the soup. Add alphabet noodles to soup; simmer for 10 minutes, or until pasta is al dente. Remove skin from cooked chicken. Remove meat from bone. Cut meat into bite-size pieces. Return meat to soup; heat through. Serve hot.

Serves 6

Nutritive Information per Serving
Calories:              192
Protein (g):            13
Fat (g):                 1
Carbohydrates (g):      26

---

# DINNER RECIPES

### Apple Rum Turkey Fillets

1 1/4 cups apple juice
2 tsp rum extract
4–6 oz turkey fillets
2 tsp honey
1 tbsp cornstarch
2 tbsp cold water
1 apple, cut into wedges

Combine 1/2 cup apple juice, 1 tsp rum, and salt and pepper to taste in a bowl. Pour marinade over turkey in a shallow dish, cover, and marinate 2 hours in refrigerator. Prepare grill or turn on broiler. Grill turkey fillets about 5 minutes per side or until cooked throughout. Combine remaining apple juice and rum in a saucepan over medium heat. Stir in honey and bring to a boil. Stir cornstarch into cold water and add to boiling liquid, stirring constantly until well blended. Cook 1 minute. Drizzle apple rum sauce over each turkey fillet. Garnish with fresh apple wedges.

Serves 1

Nutritive Information per Serving
Calories:              284
Protein (g):            42
Fat (g):                 1
Carbohydrates (g):      20

### Baked Cod

1 1/2 lb cod fillets, or other whitefish
1 tbsp plus 1 tsp olive oil
1/4 tsp lemon pepper

Preheat oven to 375°F. Arrange fillets in a baking dish. Drizzle with oil and season with salt and lemon pepper to taste. Bake 10–12 minutes, or until fish is opaque throughout.

Serves 4

Nutritive Information per Serving
Calories:              179
Protein (g):            30
Fat (g):                 6
Carbohydrates (g):      30

### Barbecued Chicken Breasts

4 skinless chicken breast halves, with bone
1/3 cup apricot preserves
2 tbsp plus 2 tsp lite soy sauce
2 tbsp plus 2 tsp ketchup
2 tsp brown sugar

Prepare grill. Place chicken on grill over medium heat. Cook 10 minutes, turning occasionally. Combine remaining ingredients in a bowl and mix well. Generously brush chicken with apricot glaze and cook 10–15 minutes longer, turning pieces often and brushing with glaze frequently until chicken is cooked throughout.

Serves 4

Nutritive Information per Serving
| | |
|---|---|
| Calories: | 290 |
| Protein (g): | 43 |
| Fat (g): | |
| Carbohydrates (g): | 23 |

## Pork Filet with Mustard-Peppercorn Sauce

1 tsp vegetable oil
4 pork filets, or boneless pork rib-end steak, 3/4 in.
1/3 cup dry white wine
1 tbsp Dijon mustard
2 tsp brined green peppercorns, drained
1/2 tsp Worcestershire sauce

Heat oil in a heavy nonstick skillet over medium-high heat. Sauté pork 3–4 minutes per side, until just cooked throughout. Remove pork from skillet and keep warm. Add wine to skillet and bring to a boil, scraping up any browned bits. Add remaining ingredients. Cook and stir 1 minute. Pour sauce over pork to serve.

Serves 4

Nutritive Information per Serving
| | |
|---|---|
| Calories: | 101 |
| Protein (g): | 13 |
| Fat (g): | 4 |
| Carbohydrates (g): | 13 |

## Cod with Orange Sauce

4 4-oz cod fillets
1/2 cup orange juice

1/2 tsp thyme, or 1 tsp fresh, chopped
1/2 tsp orange zest
1/8 tsp salt optional

Preheat oven to 375°F. Arrange cod fillets in a shallow baking dish. Pour orange juice over cod and sprinkle with thyme, orange zest, salt and pepper to taste. Bake 12–15 minutes until fish is opaque throughout. Spoon orange sauce over fish and serve.

Serves 4

Nutritive Information per Serving
| | |
|---|---|
| Calories: | 108 |
| Protein (g): | 20 |
| Fat (g): | 1 |
| Carbohydrates (g): | 4 |

## *Grill Machine Cajun Chicken Breasts*

4 boneless chicken breast halves
2 tsp olive oil
2 tsp Cajun blended spice mix
1 tbsp parsley, chopped

Preheat grill machine. Place chicken between two sheets of plastic wrap and pound lightly with a mallet or other heavy flat object to flatten slightly. Brush both sides of chicken with oil and sprinkle with spice. Place chicken on hot grill. Close cover and cook 2–3 minutes until chicken is cooked throughout. Serve sprinkled with parsley.

Serves 4

Nutritive Information per Serving
| | |
|---|---|
| Calories: | 224 |
| Protein (g): | 42 |
| Fat (g): | 5 |
| Carbohydrates (g): | 1 |

## Pasta and Salmon Salad

1/2 lb small shell pasta
1/2 lb canned salmon, drained and flaked, bones discarded
1 green bell pepper, seeded and chopped
2/3 cup celery, thinly sliced
1/2 cup red onion, chopped
3/4 cup fat-free honey Dijon salad dressing

Cook pasta in a large pan of boiling water 8–10 minutes, or until al dente. Drain, rinse under cold water, and drain again. Combine pasta, salmon, and next three ingredients in a bowl. Pour dressing over salad and toss gently.

Serves 4

Nutritive Information per Serving
Calories: 321
Protein (g): 19
Fat (g): 5
Carbohydrates (g): 49

## Roast Pork

1 lb boneless pork sirloin roast
1 clove garlic, minced
1 tsp rosemary, crushed, or 1 tbsp fresh, chopped

Preheat oven to 350°F. Place pork in a shallow roasting pan. Rub with garlic and rosemary. Season with salt and pepper to taste. Roast 25 minutes per pound or until meat thermometer registers 160°F. Remove from heat and let stand 5 minutes before carving.

Serves 6

Nutritive Information per Serving
Calories: 161
Protein (g): 25
Fat (g): 6
Carbohydrates (g): 1

## Speedy Poached Flounder

1/2 cup white wine
1/4 tsp pepper
1/4 tsp dill weed
1 1/4 lb flounder fillets

Combine all ingredients, except flounder, in a heavy skillet over medium-high heat. As soon as mixture boils, add fish. Reduce heat to medium low and gently simmer 6–8 minutes, or until fish flakes easily.

Serves 4

Nutritive Information per Serving
Calories:                    150
Protein (g):                 27
Fat (g):                      2
Carbohydrates (g):            1

## Stuffed Chicken Breasts

4 sun-dried tomatoes, packed in oil or dried
1 tsp lemon zest, grated
1 tbsp plus 1 tsp unsalted butter
2 tbsp parsley, minced
1/8 tsp salt optional
1 lb boneless skinless chicken breast halves

If using oil-packed tomatoes, drain and finely chop. If using dried tomatoes, cover tomatoes with boiling water in a bowl. Let stand 5 minutes. Drain and finely chop. Place 2 tbsp chopped tomatoes and half the lemon zest in a small bowl. Add butter, parsley, and salt. Mix thoroughly and set aside. Combine remaining tomatoes and zest in another bowl and mix thoroughly.

Using a sharp knife, cut horizontally through the center of each chicken breast to form a pocket. Do not cut all the way through. Divide tomato and lemon zest mixture into equal portions and spread in pocket of each chicken breast. Turn on broiler. Arrange chicken on a broiler pan and place 4 in. from heat source. Broil 5 minutes. Turn and broil another 4 minutes. Spread tomato and butter mixture over chicken breasts. Broil another 1–2 minutes, or until chicken is opaque throughout.

Serves 1

Nutritive Information per Serving
Calories:              166
Protein (g):            26
Fat (g):                 6
Carbohydrates (g):       1

### *Veal Cutlets*

4 4-oz veal top round steaks
1 tsp olive oil
1 tsp unsalted butter

Place veal between two sheets of wax paper and pound lightly with a mallet or other heavy flat object to flatten to about 1/4 in. thickness. Heat a heavy nonstick skillet over medium-high heat. Add oil and butter. When hot, sauté veal, in batches if necessary, about 30 seconds per side, until browned. Transfer to a serving dish. Sprinkle with salt and pepper to taste. Serve immediately.

Serves 4

Nutritive Information per Serving
Calories:              150
Protein (g):            23
Fat (g):                 6
Carbohydrates (g):       0

### *Lemon and Sage Turkey Fillets*

4 4-oz turkey breast fillets
1/4 cup fresh lemon juice
1 tsp Dijon mustard

1/4 tsp cayenne, or to taste
2/3 cup olive oil
1/4 cup dried sage, crumbled
1 lemon, cut into wedges

Place turkey between two sheets of plastic wrap and pound lightly with a mallet or other heavy flat object to flatten to 1/4 in. Combine next four ingredients and salt to taste in a jar with a tight fitting lid. Shake vigorously until emulsified, and stir in sage. Place turkey in a glass dish and cover with mustard mixture. Cover dish and marinate 25 minutes. Remove turkey and pat dry. Discard marinade. Heat a heavy nonstick skillet over medium-high heat. Sauté turkey 2 minutes per side or until just cooked throughout. Serve with lemon wedges.

Serves 1

Nutritive Information per Serving
| | |
|---|---|
| Calories: | 145 |
| Protein (g): | 29 |
| Fat (g): | 2 |
| Carbohydrates (g): | 6 |

### *Lemon Dijon Chicken*

3 1/2 tbsp lemon juice
3/4 tsp Dijon mustard
2 cloves garlic, crushed
1 1/3 cups low-sodium chicken broth, fat skimmed off top and
    discarded
4 6-oz boneless skinless chicken breast halves, washed and patted
    dry
1/4 tsp lemon pepper
2 tsp cornstarch
1/4 tsp fresh rosemary
3/4 tsp lemon peel, shredded

Combine first three ingredients and 1/3 cup chicken broth. Mix well. Pour marinade over chicken breasts and marinate in refrigerater 1 hour. Preheat broiler. Remove chicken from marinade and reserve marinade. Sprinkle chicken with lemon pepper. Broil about 10 minutes per side, or until cooked throughout.

Measure out 1 tbsp plus 1 tsp of remaining chicken broth and set aside. Combine rest of chicken broth with the marinade in a saucepan. Bring to a boil and then reduce heat to low. Simmer 15 minutes.

Mix together cornstarch and reserved chicken broth. Blend into simmering mixture and cook 5 minutes longer. Strain the sauce through a china cap or fine sieve. Add rosemary and lemon peel. Serve sauce over chicken.

Serves 4

Nutritive Information per Serving
Calories:              208
Protein (g):            41
Fat (g):                 3
Carbohydrates (g):       4

### *Mustard Grilled Turkey Breasts*

2 tbsp Dijon mustard
2 cloves garlic, minced
1/2 tsp rosemary
1/4 tsp pepper
1 tbsp virgin olive oil
4 4-oz turkey breast fillets

Prepare grill or broiler. Combine all ingredients, except turkey, in a jar with a tight-fitting lid. Shake vigorously. Grill or broil turkey breasts 4 minutes per side. Spread half the mustard mixture over one side of turkey breasts and grill or broil 3 minutes. Turn and coat with remaining mustard mixture. Broil another 3 minutes, or until turkey is cooked throughout.

Serves 4

Nutritive Information per Serving
Calories:                165
Protein (g):              28
Fat (g):                   5
Carbohydrates (g):         2

### *Penne with Chicken, Peas, and Peppers*

2 1/2 cups penne or other tube pasta
1/2 cup chicken stock
1 cup frozen green peas, thawed
1 tbsp olive oil
1 clove garlic, minced
1 red bell pepper, seeded and diced
3/4 lb boneless skinless chicken breast halves, cut into 1/2 in. pieces
1/4 cup Romano or parmesan cheese, grated

Cook pasta in a large pan of boiling water 10 minutes, or until al
dente. Drain and set aside. Combine stock and 1/2 cup peas in a
food processor or blender and process until smooth. Set aside.
Heat oil in a heavy nonstick skillet over medium-high heat. Sauté
garlic 30 seconds. Add bell pepper and chicken and sauté 4 minutes, stirring occasionally, or until chicken is cooked throughout.
Add pea purée, whole peas, and salt and pepper to taste. Stir well.
Stir in pasta and bring to a boil. Cook 2 minutes, or until mixture
thickens, stirring constantly. Stir in cheese and toss well before
serving.

Serves 1

Nutritive Information per Serving
Calories:                373
Protein (g):              30
Fat (g):                   6
Carbohydrates (g):        47

## *Pan-Fried Red Snapper*

2/3 cup seasoned breadcrumbs
1 1/4 lb red snapper fillets
1 tbsp plus 1 tsp oil
1 1/4 lemons or limes, cut in wedges

Place breadcrumbs in a shallow plate and dredge snapper to coat. Heat oil in a heavy nonstick skillet over medium heat. Cook 5–6 minutes per side until fish flakes. Serve with lemon or lime wedges.

Serves 4

Nutritive Information per Serving
Calories:            265
Protein (g):         32
Fat (g):             7
Carbohydrates (g):    17

## *Peachy Pork Picante*

1 lb boneless pork, cut into 3/4 in. cubes
1 tbsp taco seasoning
1 tsp vegetable oil
1 cup chunky style prepared salsa
1/3 cup peach preserves

Coat pork cubes with taco seasoning. Heat oil in a heavy nonstick skillet over medium-high heat. Sauté pork 2–3 minutes, stirring occasionally until browned on all sides. Add salsa and preserves. Reduce heat to low, cover and simmer 15–20 minutes.

Serves 4

Nutritive Information per Serving
Calories:            253
Protein (g):         26
Fat (g):             7
Carbohydrates (g):    20

## Slow Cooker Turkey Tortilla Soup

2 skinless turkey thighs
1 lb canned diced tomatoes
1 onion, diced
1 clove garlic, crushed
1 jalapeño pepper, seeded and chopped (wear rubber gloves)
4 cups chicken stock
4 corn tortillas, cut into 1/4 in. slices
1/2 cup fresh cilantro, chopped

Combine first five ingredients and salt to taste in slow cooker. Cover and cook on low 7–8 hours, until turkey is tender. Preheat oven to 400°F. Arrange tortilla strips in a single layer on a baking sheet. Bake 6–8 minutes, stirring occasionally, until golden. Set aside. Remove turkey from slow cooker and cool slightly. Remove and discard bones. Chop turkey meat and divide among soup bowls. Process remaining soup mixture in a blender or food processor until puréed. Pour over turkey in soup bowls. Serve sprinkled with tortilla strips and cilantro.

Serves 6

Nutritive Information per Serving
Calories:             215
Protein (g):           28
Fat (g):                4
Carbohydrates (g):     17

## Grilled Shrimp with Pasta and Pineapple Salsa

From the American Diabetes Association's *Flavorful Seasons Cookbook*

2 lb pineapple chunks, packed in their own juice, drained
1 large red bell pepper, chopped
1 large red onion, chopped
1 jalapeño pepper, minced
1/2 cup orange juice

1/3 cup lime juice
1 1/2 cups shrimp, peeled and deveined
6 cups cooked rotini pasta

In a large bowl, combine all salsa ingredients, except the shrimp and pasta. Prepare an outside grill with an oiled rack set 4 in. above the heat source. On a gas grill, set the heat to high. Grill the shrimp on each side for 2 minutes. Toss the pasta with the salsa, arrange the shrimp on top, and serve.

Serves 6

Nutritive Information per Serving
Calories:              301
Protein (g):            14
Fat (g):                 2
Carbohydrates (g):      59

### *Halibut in Foil*

From the American Diabetes Association's *Diabetic Meals in 30 Minutes or Less*

2 tsp olive oil
6 4-oz halibut steaks
1/2 cup dry white wine
6 thyme sprigs
6 lemon slices
1 1/2 tsp fennel seeds
6 fresh parsley sprigs
fresh ground pepper

Preheat oven to 350°F. Tear aluminum foil into six large squares. Brush each square with some olive oil. Place the halibut in the center of the square. Drizzle each steak with some of the wine. Put a thyme sprig, lemon slice, a few fennel seeds, and a parsley sprig on each piece of fish. Grind pepper over each piece of fish. Seal the foil into a packet. Place all packets on a baking sheet and bake for

10–15 minutes. Place a packet on each plate, and let each person carefully open the packet. Pour all juices on top of the fish.

Serves 6

Nutritive Information per Serving
Calories:                 265
Protein (g):               32
Fat (g):                    7
Carbohydrates (g):         17

### Turkey Provençal

From the American Diabetes Association's *Diabetic Meals in 30 Minutes or Less*

1 1/2 lb turkey fillets
2 tbsp unbleached white flour
salt and pepper
2 tsp olive oil
1 onion, diced
2 cloves garlic, minced
1 1/2 cups canned crushed tomatoes
1 tbsp fresh rosemary, chopped
1 tbsp fresh thyme, chopped
1/4 cup sliced black olives
2 tsp capers
1/2 cup fresh parsley, minced

In a Ziploc bag, place the turkey fillets with the flour, salt, and pepper. Shake the bag until the turkey fillets are coated with flour. In a large skillet over medium heat, heat the oil. Add the turkey fillets and sauté on each side for 4 minutes. Remove from the skillet. In the same skillet, sauté the onion and garlic for 5 minutes until the onions begin to brown. Add the crushed tomatoes. Bring to a boil. Lower the heat and let simmer for 5 minutes. Add the turkey, rosemary, thyme, olives, and capers to the skillet. Simmer over low heat for 10 minutes. Add the parsley and serve.

Serves 6

Nutritive Information per Serving
Calories:              183
Protein (g):            29
Fat (g):                 3
Carbohydrates (g):       9

### *Chicken Casserole*

2 tbsp butter
4 chicken breast halves, boneless and skinless, and sliced into 1 in.
    strips
1 cup chopped onion
2 cups chicken stock
1/2 cup mushrooms, sliced or quartered
2 tbsp fresh chopped parsley, divided
2 cup peas
1 1/2 cups whole baby carrots, cooked
2 tbsp cornstarch
2 tbsp cool water

In a large frying pan, using medium heat, melt butter and sauté the
chicken and onions until golden brown. Add the chicken stock,
mushrooms, and 1 tbsp of the chopped parsley; season with salt
and pepper. Cover and simmer for 10 minutes, adding the peas
and cooked carrots and cooking for an additional 5 minutes.
Remove the chicken and vegetables from the frying pan and place
in large serving bowl; leave the cooking liquids in the pan. Mix
cornstarch and water in a small mixing bowl, then add to cooking
liquid in frying pan; cook until mixture thickens. Pour thickened
sauce over chicken mixture; garnish with remaining parsley.

Serves 4

Nutritive Information per Serving
Calories:              300
Protein (g):            32

Fat (g):                          9
Carbohydrates (g):      22

### *Chicken Divan*

1 cup uncooked pasta
1 whole cooked chicken breast, boneless and skinless

*Mornay Sauce*
2 tbsp butter
2 tbsp flour
1 cup and 2 tbsp chicken stock
1 tbsp sherry
1/4 cup skim milk
1 egg, slightly beaten
1/4 cup grated parmesan cheese
2 cups broccoli, cut into florets
paprika, to taste

Cook pasta according to package directions; set aside. Thinly slice chicken breast; set aside.

Make Mornay sauce: melt butter in a medium-size saucepan over a medium heat; whisk in flour. Gradually whisk in chicken stock, sherry, and milk. Cook until mixture comes to a boil; boil for 1 minute. Gradually whisk about 1/4 of the chicken stock mixture into the egg. Then, gradually whisk the egg mixture back into the warm sauce in the saucepan. Whisk in parmesan cheese.

Assemble as follows: Place the cooked pasta in the bottom of an 8 by 8 by 2 in. or 9 by 9 by 2 in. baking pan. Place broccoli around the edges of the pan on top of the pasta. Place the sliced chicken in the center of the pan, covering the pasta. Pour Mornay sauce over the top of all the ingredients. Sprinkle with paprika. Bake at 400°F for about 20 minutes till cooked through.

Serves 4

Nutritive Information per Serving
Calories:                       305

| Protein (g): | 24 |
|---|---|
| Fat (g): | 11 |
| Carbohydrates (g): | 28 |

### *Chicken Provencal*

1 tbsp butter
4 chicken breast halves, skinned, boned, and butterflied
1 tbsp butter
1 tomato, peeled and chopped
1 onion, chopped
1/2 cup chicken stock
1/2 tsp minced garlic
2 tsp fresh parsley, chopped
1 tsp fresh thyme, chopped
salt, to taste
black pepper, to taste
6 black olives, sliced

Heat a large frying pan to medium or medium high; add 1 tbsp butter. Sauté the chicken breasts in the melted butter till cooked through (about 6 minutes). Remove from pan; set aside. Add 1 tbsp butter to the same pan and then sauté tomatoes and onion until just tender; add chicken stock. Cook until sauce is reduced to about 1/2 the original quantity. Season tomato mixture with garlic, parsley, thyme, salt, and black pepper. Place tomato mixture on plate; top with chicken; garnish with black olives.

Serves 4

Nutritive Information per Serving
| Calories: | 217 |
|---|---|
| Protein (g): | 28 |
| Fat (g): | 9 |
| Carbohydrates (g): | 5 |

## *Chicken Vegetable Stir Fry*

1 tsp garlic
1 tsp cornstarch
4 tsp soy sauce, low sodium
2 tbsp vermouth
4 chicken breast halves, boneless and skinless
3 carrots, peeled, and cut julienne
2 stalks celery, sliced diagonally
2 cups broccoli, chopped
1 can water chestnuts, sliced
2 tbsp oil, divided
1/2 tsp ginger
2 tbsp soy sauce, low sodium
2 tbsp cornstarch
1/2 cup cold water

Prepare marinade by mixing garlic, 1 tsp cornstarch, 4 tsp soy sauce, and vermouth together in a medium-size bowl; set aside. Slice, across the grain, chicken breasts into 1/4 in. strips. Mix with marinade. Refrigerate. Heat a large frying pan over medium-high heat. Add 1 tbsp oil. Add vegetables and water chestnuts to hot oil. Sauté till crisp and tender. Remove from pan; set aside. Add 1 tbsp oil to the same pan. Sauté chicken until cooked through. Add vegetables to chicken; heat through. Mix 2 tbsp cornstarch with 2 tbsp soy sauce, then stir in water and ginger. Add to frying pan. Cook till sauce thickens.

Serves 4

Nutritive Information per Serving
Calories:                    294
Protein (g):                  30
Fat (g):                      10
Carbohydrates (g):            16

Note: 1 lb of peeled, deveined shrimp may be substituted in this recipe for the chicken.

Nutritional Information per Serving (Shrimp)
Calories:                286
Protein (g):              31
Fat (g):                   8
Carbohydrates (g):        18

### *Chicken with Lemon Thyme Sauce*

1/4 cup flour
1/2 tsp salt
1/2 tsp pepper
4 chicken breast halves, boneless and skinless
2 tbsp olive oil, divided
1 tbsp butter
1 cup onion, coarsely chopped
1 cup chicken stock
3 tbsp lemon juice, divided
1/2 tsp thyme
1 tbsp capers
2 tbsp chopped parsley
1 lemon, thinly sliced, for garnish, optional

In a large plastic bag, mix the flour, salt, and pepper. Add chicken and shake to coat lightly. Remove chicken; set aside. Reserve the extra seasoned flour. Heat a large frying pan over a medium heat. Add 1 tbsp of oil. Sauté chicken 5 minutes until browned. Add the remaining 1 tbsp oil. Turn chicken and brown an additional 5 minutes. Place chicken on a plate; set aside.

Add butter to frying pan. Sauté onion in butter for 2–3 minutes until it softens. Use a wire whisk to stir reserved flour mixture into onion mixture. Cook about 1 minute. Whisk chicken stock, 2 tbsp lemon juice, and thyme into onion mixture; bring to a boil while whisking constantly.

Return chicken to frying pan, reduce heat to medium low and cover. Cook until chicken is cooked through (5–10 minutes). Place chicken on serving plate. Stir in remaining 1 tbsp lemon juice and capers. Pour sauce over chicken; sprinkle with parsley; garnish with lemon slices if desired.

Serves 4

Nutritive Information per Serving

| | |
|---|---|
| Calories: | 239 |
| Protein (g): | 28 |
| Fat (g): | 13 |
| Carbohydrates (g): | 6 |

### *Crab Louis*

2 cups salad greens, bite size, and chilled
1 egg, hard cooked, peeled, and sliced
1 tomato, cut into wedges
6 black olives
3 oz crabmeat, drained and cartilage removed
2 tbsp Thousand Island dressing, lowfat

Place greens on a salad plate. Arrange egg, tomato, and black olives around edges of plate. Place crabmeat in the center of the lettuce. Serve dressing on the side.

Serves 1

Nutritive Information per Serving

| | |
|---|---|
| Calories: | 258 |
| Protein (g): | 19 |
| Fat (g): | 10 |
| Carbohydrates (g): | 12 |

Note: 3 oz cooked, peeled, and deveined shrimp may be substituted for the crab.

Nutritional Information per Serving (Shrimp)

| | |
|---|---|
| Calories: | 290 |
| Protein (g): | 28 |
| Fat (g): | 9 |
| Carbohydrates (g): | 13 |

## *Crystal Shrimp with Sweet and Sour Sauce*

1/2 cup sweet and sour sauce
1/2 cup water
2 tsp cornstarch
1 egg white, slightly beaten
1/2 lb medium-size raw shrimp, peeled, and deveined
2 tbsp oil, divided
1/2 tsp minced garlic
2 carrots, cut diagonally into thin slices
1 green bell pepper, cut into thin strips
1 cup chopped onion
1 tbsp sesame seed, toasted

Blend sweet and sour sauce with water; set aside. Measure cornstarch into large plastic bag. Coat shrimp with egg white; shake off excess. Add shrimp to cornstarch in bag; shake bag to coat shrimp. Heat a large frying pan over a medium-high heat. Add 1 tbsp oil. Add garlic then immediately add shrimp and stir-fry 2 minutes until shrimp are pink. Remove from pan; set aside. Heat additional 1 tbsp oil in same pan over medium-high heat. Add carrots, green pepper, and onion; stir-fry for 4 minutes. Add shrimp and sweet and sour sauce to carrot mixture. Cook and stir until all ingredients are coated with sauce. Remove from heat and sprinkle with sesame seeds. Serve immediately.

Serves 4

Nutritive Information per Serving
Calories:                    231
Protein (g):                  18
Fat (g):                       8
Carbohydrates (g):            22

Note: Recipe may be made with 1/2 lb boneless, skinless chicken breast, cut into bite size pieces.

Nutritive Information per Serving (Chicken breast)
Calories:                    226
Protein (g):                  14

Fat (g):                     9
Carbohydrates (g):      21

### Grilled Chicken Breasts

This recipe can be used in a variety of ways (in chicken divan, with spaghetti sauce, on Caesar salad, and so on).

4 chicken breast halves, boneless and skinless
2 tbsp lemon juice or white wine
1 tbsp olive oil

*Seasoning* (select one of the following choices):
lemon pepper, to taste
equal parts of thyme, oregano, and basil, to taste
paprika, to taste
garlic and black pepper, to taste

Combine lemon juice or white wine and olive oil in a large plastic bag. Add your choice of seasoning. Shake to combine. Add chicken to the bag. Marinate in the refrigerator for 30 minutes. Heat grill to high. Place marinated chicken on grill; turn once after 3–4 minutes. Cook through (time will vary depending on grill temperature).

Serves 4

Nutritive Information per Serving
Calories:                  172
Protein (g):                27
Fat (g):                     7
Carbohydrates (g):      <1

### Lemon Chicken

2 tbsp butter
2 tbsp olive oil
4 chicken breast halves, boneless and skinless
1 tbsp flour

1 cup chicken stock
1 egg
2 tbsp lemon juice
salt and pepper to taste

Heat a large frying pan over a medium-high heat. Add butter and olive oil. Sauté chicken until golden. Sprinkle flour into frying pan. Cook and stir for 3 minutes. Add chicken stock. Cover and simmer for 15 minutes, until chicken is tender and cooked through. Remove chicken and set aside. In a medium-size bowl, whisk egg and lemon juice together. Slowly whisk about 1/4 of the pan mixture into the egg mixture. Then, whisk the egg mixture into the remaining ingredients in the pan. Return the chicken to the pan. Reduce heat to low and heat for 2 minutes, or until heated through.

Serves 4

Nutritive Information per Serving
Calories:               282
Protein (g):             29
Fat (g):                 17
Carbohydrates (g):        2

### Red Chicken with Almonds

1/4 cup flour
1/2 tsp salt
1/2 tsp thyme
1/4 tsp pepper
4 chicken breast halves, boneless and skinless
2 tbsp oil
1 cup chopped onion
2 tsp paprika
1/2 tsp minced garlic
8 oz tomatoes, cut up and undrained
1/2 cup water
1/4 cup toasted almonds

In a large plastic bag, combine the flour, salt, thyme, and pepper. Add chicken and shake to coat; set aside. Heat a large frying pan over a medium heat. Add oil to pan and then flour the coated chicken. Cook until chicken is lightly browned. Add onion, paprika, garlic, and cook for 5 minutes. Stir in tomatoes and water; cover and cook about 15 minutes until chicken is cooked through. Sprinkle with almonds.

Serves 4

Nutritive Information per Serving
Calories:                   305
Protein (g):                 31
Fat (g):                     15
Carbohydrates (g):           13

### Shrimp Rémoulade

1 lb shrimp, cooked, peeled, and deveined
8 cups mixed greens
4 plum tomatoes, thinly sliced

*Rémoulade Sauce*
2 tsp paprika
4 tsp country Dijon mustard
2 tsp ketchup
2 tsp horseradish
3 tbsp celery, finely chopped
4 tsp onion, finely chopped
1/4 tsp sugar
1/4 tsp tabasco
2 tsp fresh parsley, finely chopped
1/3 cup corn oil

1. Make rémoulade sauce: in a small mixing bowl, place all ingredients, except oil; combine using a wire whisk. Pour the oil into the bowl in a steady stream while constantly whisking the ingredients to form an emulsion.

Shrimp may be added to rémoulade sauce 2–3 hours before serving to intensify flavor, if desired. Place lettuce on individual plates, place shrimp and sauce on top; garnish with sliced tomatoes. Serve chilled.

Serves 4

Nutritive Information per Serving
Calories:                          330
Protein (g):                       31
Fat (g):                           20
Carbohydrates (g):                 10

---

# Vegetable Sides

### Broccoli with Italian Dressing

1 lb broccoli florets
2 tbsp fat-free Italian dressing

Place broccoli in a steamer basket over boiling water. Cover saucepan and steam 4–5 minutes, or until bright green and almost tender. Drain. Combine with dressing and season with salt and pepper to taste.

Serves 4

Nutritive Information per Serving
Calories:                          34
Protein (g):                       3
Fat (g):                           .4
Carbohydrates (g):                 6

### Baked Potatoes

4 baking potatoes, scrubbed
1/2 cup nonfat sour cream

Preheat oven to 400°F. Bake potatoes 45 minutes, or until tender.

Serve potatoes topped with a dollop of fat-free sour cream and seasoned with salt and pepper to taste.

Serves 4

Nutritive Information per Serving
Calories:              168
Protein (g):             5
Fat (g):                .1
Carbohydrates (g):      37

### Asparagus with Italian Dressing

1 lb asparagus, tough ends discarded
1/4 cup fat-free Italian dressing

Place asparagus in a steamer basket over boiling water. Cover saucepan and steam 5–7 minutes, or until asparagus is tender. Rinse under cold water. Drain thoroughly and toss with dressing.

Serves 4

Nutritive Information per Serving
Calories:               31
Protein (g):             3
Fat (g):                .2
Carbohydrates (g):       6

### Cooked Peppers and Mushrooms

1/4 cup chicken stock or water
1 tsp unsalted butter
1 large red bell pepper, cored, seeded, and cut into 1 in. squares
1 yellow or green bell pepper, cored, seeded, and cut into 1 in. squares
1/2 lb mushrooms, sliced
1/2 tsp tarragon, or 2 tbsp fresh, chopped
1/8 tsp salt optional
1 tbsp parmesan cheese

Heat stock and butter in a heavy nonstick skillet over medium heat. Sauté bell peppers and mushrooms 7–8 minutes, or until mushrooms are tender. Stir in tarragon and season with salt and pepper to taste. Cook another minute. Sprinkle with cheese.

Serves 4

Nutritive Information per Serving
Calories:               44
Protein (g):             3
Fat (g):                 2
Carbohydrates (g):       6

### *Lowfat Vegetable Stew*

2 tbsp water
1 cup zucchini, thinly sliced
1 1/4 cups yellow squash, thinly sliced
1/2 cup green bell pepper, cut into 2 in. strips
1/4 cup celery, cut into 2 in. strips
1/4 cup onion, chopped
1/2 tsp caraway seeds
1/8 tsp garlic powder
1 medium tomato, cut into 8 wedges

Add first six ingredients to a heavy nonstick skillet over medium heat. Cover and cook 4 minutes, or until vegetables are just tender. Add remaining ingredients, reduce heat to low, cover, and cook another 2 minutes.

Serves 4

Nutritive Information per Serving
Calories:               38
Protein (g):             2
Fat (g):                 1
Carbohydrates (g):       9

## Steamed Cabbage

1 1/4 lb cabbage, cut into wedges
1 tsp unsalted butter, melted

Place cabbage in a steamer basket over boiling water. Cover
saucepan and steam 8–10 minutes, or until cabbage is bright green
and tender. Do not overcook. Remove cabbage from steamer.
Drizzle with melted butter. Season with salt and pepper to taste.

Serves 4

Nutritive Information per Serving
Calories:                40
Protein (g):              2
Fat (g):                  2
Carbohydrates (g):        6

## Stuffed Bell Peppers

2 small green bell peppers
2 tsp vegetable oil
1/8 tsp mustard seeds
2 cups shredded cabbage
1/4 cup carrots, grated
1/8 tsp turmeric
1/2 tsp salt
1/2 tsp coriander
1/8 tsp cayenne pepper (optional)

Wash and dry the bell peppers. Cut the bell peppers lengthwise in
half. Remove the seeds and cut out the pulp part near the stem,
leaving the pepper in a cuplike form. Set aside. Heat 1/2 tsp olive
oil in a large, nonstick fry pan over medium heat. Add mustard
seeds, covering with a lid to avoid splattering. Fry for a few seconds
until the mustard seeds stop popping. Add the shredded cabbage
and carrots. Stir. Add turmeric, salt, coriander, and cayenne pepper
and stir. Cover with a lid, heat through, reduce heat and simmer
for 5–7 minutes. The vegetables should be slightly tender. If there

is any excess liquid accumulated at the bottom of the pan, increase heat to evaporate it. Remove from the heat and cool to room temperature. Divide cabbage mixture into eight equal parts. Stuff the bell pepper halves with the mixture.

Clean the fry pan and heat the remaining 1 1/2 tsp oil over medium heat. Place the stuffed bell peppers in the hot oil with the stuffed side facing up. Reduce heat, cover with a lid and simmer for 10–12 minutes until the bell peppers become tender. The bottom of the bell peppers will be slightly black. Transfer the bell peppers to a serving tray.

Serves 4

Nutritive Information per Serving
Calories:               40
Protein (g):             1
Fat (g):                 3
Carbohydrates (g):       5

### *Broccoli with Lemon*

1 1/4 lb broccoli florets
2 tbsp lemon juice

Place broccoli in a steamer basket over boiling water. Cover pan and steam 5–7 minutes, or until tender. Toss with lemon juice before serving.

Serves 4

Nutritive Information per Serving
Calories:               42
Protein (g):             4
Fat (g):                .5
Carbohydrates (g):       8

### *Steamed Carrots*

1 1/2 lb carrots, peeled and sliced
1 tsp unsalted butter

Place carrots in a steamer basket over boiling water. Cover saucepan and steam 5–7 minutes, or until carrots are tender. Drain and transfer to a serving bowl. Add butter and salt and pepper to taste.

Serves 4

Nutritive Information per Serving
Calories:            85
Protein (g):          2
Fat (g):             1
Carbohydrates (g):   18

### Green Beans in Mustard

1 lb green beans, trimmed
1 tsp unsalted butter or margarine
1 tbsp plus 1 tsp coarse mustard
1/4 tsp salt, optional

Place beans in a steamer basket over boiling water. Cover saucepan and steam 5–7 minutes, or until tender. Melt butter in a heavy nonstick skillet over medium heat. Stir in mustard. Add green beans and toss to coat. Season with salt and pepper to taste.

Serves 4

Nutritive Information per Serving
Calories:            48
Protein (g):          2
Fat (g):             1
Carbohydrates (g):    8

### Maple Beans

2 tbsp plus 2 tsp maple syrup
1 1/2 tbsp dark rum
1 1/2 tsp ketchup
1 tsp Dijon mustard

1/2 onion, chopped
1 lb canned baked beans
1/4 cup real bacon pieces

Prepare broiler. Whisk first four ingredients together in a heavy saucepan. Add onion and beans, and bring to a boil over high heat. Reduce heat to medium and simmer 10–12 minutes, until sauce is thickened. Transfer beans to a baking dish and top with bacon pieces. Broil 2 minutes about 5 in. from heat source.

Serves 4

Nutritive Information per Serving
Calories:               188
Protein (g):              9
Fat (g):                  2
Carbohydrates (g):       35

### *Creamy Carrots and Peas*

3/4 lb carrots, thinly sliced
1/2 lb green peas, thawed if frozen
1 oz breakfast cheese, cut into cubes and softened
1/4 tsp white pepper

Place carrots in a steamer basket over boiling water. Cover saucepan and steam 4 minutes. Add peas and steam 3–4 minutes, or until peas are tender. Drain and return vegetables to saucepan. Add remaining ingredients and salt to taste and toss.

Serves 4

Nutritive Information per Serving
Calories:               102
Protein (g):              5
Fat (g):                  2
Carbohydrates (g):       17

### Buttered Green Beans

1 1/2 lb green beans, trimmed
2 tsp unsalted butter, melted

Place green beans in a steamer basket over boiling water. Cover saucepan and steam 8–10 minutes, or until tender. Transfer to a serving bowl and toss with butter and salt and pepper to taste.

Serves 4

Nutritive Information per Serving
Calories:                   70
Protein (g):                 3
Fat (g):                     2
Carbohydrates (g):          12

### Rice with Peas

2 cups water
1 cup long grain rice
1 1/2 cups green peas
2 tsp unsalted butter

Combine water, salt, and pepper to taste in a medium saucepan over high heat and bring to a boil. Stir in rice and return to a boil. Immediately reduce heat to low, cover saucepan, and simmer 10 minutes. Add peas without stirring. Cover saucepan and simmer another 8–10 minutes until rice is tender and liquid is absorbed. Add butter and fluff with a fork before serving.

Serves 4

Nutritive Information per Serving
Calories:                  225
Protein (g):                 6
Fat (g):                     3
Carbohydrates (g):          44

### Broccoli Tomatoes Sauté

2 tsp unsalted butter
1 lb broccoli florets
1 cup recipe-ready crushed tomatoes

Melt butter in a heavy saucepan over medium heat. Sauté broccoli florets 2–3 minutes. Add tomatoes and salt and pepper to taste. Cover and simmer 3–4 minutes, or until broccoli is tender.

Serves 4

Nutritive Information per Serving
Calories:              60
Protein (g):            4
Fat (g):                2
Carbohydrates (g):      9

### Golden Mashed Potatoes

1 lb potatoes, peeled and cut into 1 in. cubes
2 tsp unsalted butter
1 onion, finely chopped
1 tsp paprika
3/4 cup plain lowfat yogurt
1/8 tsp salt optional

Place potatoes in a steamer basket over boiling water. Cover saucepan and steam 12–15 minutes, or until tender. Melt butter in a heavy nonstick skillet over medium heat. Sauté onions 7–8 minutes, or until golden. Remove from heat and stir in paprika. Combine potatoes, onions, yogurt, salt, and pepper to taste in a bowl. Mash potatoes thoroughly before serving.

Serves 4

Nutritive Information per Serving
Calories:             188
Protein (g):            6

Fat (g):                    3
Carbohydrates (g):     36

## Light Lemon Carrots

1 tbsp unsalted butter
1 1/2 lb carrots, peeled and cut into 1 1/2 in. sticks
1/2 tsp sugar
1/4 tsp salt optional, or to taste
1/8 tsp white pepper
1/4 cup water
3 tbsp lemon juice

Melt butter in a heavy saucepan over medium heat. Sauté carrots 3 minutes. Stir in sugar, salt, white pepper, and water, and bring to a boil. Cover saucepan and reduce heat to low. Simmer 3 minutes, or until carrots are almost tender. Stir in lemon juice and simmer uncovered over medium-high heat until carrots are glazed.

Serves 4

Nutritive Information per Serving
Calories:               107
Protein (g):              2
Fat (g):                  3
Carbohydrates (g):      19

## Tarragon Asparagus

1 1/2 lb asparagus spears, fibrous ends trimmed
1 tbsp Passover margarine
1 1/2 tbsp scallions, chopped
1 1/2 tsp fresh tarragon, snipped
1 tbsp fresh parsley
1 1/2 tsp lemon juice

Place asparagus in a steamer basket over boiling water. Cover pan and steam 5 minutes, or until tender. Do not overcook. Drain immediately. Melt margarine in a skillet over medium-high heat.

Add remaining ingredients. Spoon over asparagus and serve.

Serves 4

Nutritive Information per Serving
Calories:              53
Protein (g):            4
Fat (g):                3
Carbohydrates (g):      5

### *Curried Carrots*

1 lb carrots, peeled and cut into 1/2 in. slices
1 tbsp homestyle apricot spread
1 1/2 tsp lemon juice
3/4 tsp Dijon mustard
1 tsp curry powder
1 tsp unsalted butter
2 tsp vegetable oil
1 1/2 tsp brown sugar
1/4 cup raisins

Place carrots in a steamer basket over boiling water. Cover saucepan and steam 5–7 minutes, or until almost tender. Remove carrots from steamer and set aside. Combine apricot spread, lemon juice, mustard, and curry powder in a small bowl. Heat butter and oil in a heavy nonstick skillet over medium-high heat. When oil is hot, sauté carrots 1 minute. Stir in brown sugar and raisins, and sauté another 1–2 minutes. Add spice mixture, stirring constantly 2–3 minutes, scraping down sides of skillet, or until carrots are glazed.

Serves 4

Nutritive Information per Serving
Calories:             126
Protein (g):            2
Fat (g):                4
Carbohydrates (g):     24

## Lemon Green Beans

1 lb green beans
1/4 cup water
1/4 cup lemon juice
1 tbsp plus 1 tsp unsalted butter
1 tsp lemon zest, grated
1 tsp parsley, chopped

Place beans in a steamer basket over boiling water. Cover saucepan and steam 5–7 minutes, or until green beans are tender. Rinse under cold water and drain. Combine water and lemon juice in a heavy nonstick skillet over medium heat. Simmer 2–3 minutes, or until reduced by half. Stir in butter. Add green beans and lemon zest. Simmer 3–4 minutes, or until green beans are heated throughout. Remove from heat. Add parsley and salt to taste and toss.

Serves 4

Nutritive Information per Serving
Calories:                  73
Protein (g):                2
Fat (g):                    4
Carbohydrates (g):         10

## Chilled Potatoes in Creamy Herb Sauce

2 red potatoes, or new potatoes, unpeeled and sliced
1/2 cup frozen peas, thawed
1/4 green bell pepper, chopped
3/4 cup nonfat yogurt
1 tbsp fresh parsley, snipped
1 tbsp green onions, sliced
1/2 tsp dried basil leaves, crushed
1/8 tsp white pepper

Bring small amount of water to a boil in a saucepan. Add potatoes and cook, covered 25–30 minutes, or until tender. Drain and cool.

Slice and place in a bowl. Toss with peas and bell pepper. Add remaining ingredients and salt and pepper to taste. Toss gently to coat. Cover and chill until ready to serve.

Serves 4

Nutritive Information per Serving

Calories: 94
Protein (g): 6
Fat (g): .2
Carbohydrates (g): 20

### *Herbed Potato Salad*

10 oz red new potatoes, scrubbed
1/2 cup frozen peas, thawed
1/4 cup green bell pepper, seeded and chopped
3/4 cup nonfat plain yogurt
1 tbsp parsley
1 tbsp scallions, sliced
1/2 tsp dried basil leaves, crushed
1/8 tsp white pepper

Bring potatoes, with enough water to cover, to a boil in a heavy saucepan. Add salt to taste. Cover pan, reduce heat to medium and simmer 25–30 minutes, or until tender. Drain. Rinse under cold running water to cool. Cut into 1/4 in. slices and combine with peas and bell pepper in a bowl. Combine remaining ingredients and salt to taste and pour over potato mixture. Toss gently to coat. Cover and chill.

Serves 4

Nutritive Information per Serving

Calories: 107
Protein (g): 5
Fat (g): .2
Carbohydrates (g): 22

## Quick Vegetable Medley

2 cups frozen mixed vegetables, thawed, include broccoli, cauliflower, and carrots
2/3 cup white wine
2 tsp fresh dill, minced
3/4 tsp garlic, minced
2 tsp fresh lemon juice
salt and pepper

Combine all ingredients in a saucepan and cook over medium-
high heat for 5–6 minutes. Remove the vegetables with a slotted
spoon and keep warm. Bring the liquid remaining in the pot to a
boil. Lower the heat and reduce by 1/3. Pour over the cooked vegetables and serve.

Serves 4

Nutritive Information per Serving
Calories:           82
Protein (g):         3
Fat (g):            .1
Carbohydrates (g):  12

## Baked Spaghetti Squash

3 lb spaghetti squash, halved lengthwise and seeded

Preheat oven to 350°F. Place squash, cut side down, in a baking
dish. Add 1/2 in. of water. Bake 40–45 minutes, or until squash is
tender. Remove squash from water and cool. Remove the spaghet-
tilike strands by scraping squash with a fork.

Microwave directions: Place squash, cut side down, in a baking
dish and add 1/4 cup water. Cover the dish with heavy-duty plastic
wrap and make vent holes. Microwave at high for 15 minutes, or
about 5 minutes per pound, until squash is tender.

Serves 4

Nutritive Information per Serving

| | |
|---|---|
| Calories: | 112 |
| Protein (g): | 2 |
| Fat (g): | 2 |
| Carbohydrates (g): | 23 |

## Microwave Lemon Carrots

4 carrots, peeled and cut into 1/4 in. rounds
1 tbsp unsalted butter
1 tbsp lemon juice, or more to taste

Arrange carrots in one layer in a microwave-safe dish and dot with butter. Cover and microwave 6 minutes on high, or until almost tender. Sprinkle with lemon juice and season with salt and pepper to taste.

Serves 4

Nutritive Information per Serving

| | |
|---|---|
| Calories: | 59 |
| Protein (g): | 1 |
| Fat (g): | 3 |
| Carbohydrates (g): | 8 |

## Grilled Vegetable Basket

1/4 cup olive oil
1/4 cup balsamic vinegar
3 cloves garlic, minced
2 tsp fresh rosemary, minced
1 tsp fresh basil, minced
2 tsp lemon peel
salt and pepper
1 fennel bulb
2 Belgian endives, halved lengthwise

1 small zucchini, sliced on the diagonal into 2 in. slices
1 small red onion, sliced into 6 slices, 2 in. thick

Purée the first seven ingredients in a blender until smooth. Set aside. In a large pot of boiling water, parboil the fennel for 5 minutes. Drain. Place all the vegetables in a glass dish, cover with the marinade and marinate for 15 minutes. Prepare an outside grill with an oiled rack set 4 in. above the heat source. On a gas grill, set the heat to high. Add the vegetables to an oiled, wired-hinged vegetable basket. Grill, turning constantly, for 15–20 minutes, or until the vegetables are slightly charred.

Serves 6

Nutritive Information per Serving
| | |
|---|---|
| Calories: | 111 |
| Protein (g): | 2 |
| Fat (g): | 9 |
| Carbohydrates (g): | 8 |

### Snow Peas with Water Chestnuts and Bamboo Shoots

From the American Diabetes Association's *Diabetic Meals in 30 Minutes or Less*

2 tsp peanut oil
1/2 cup onion, diced
1/4 cup celery, diced
2 cups snow peas, trimmed
1/2 cup sliced water chestnuts
1/2 cup canned bamboo shoots, sliced
1/2 cup low-sodium lowfat chicken stock
salt and pepper

In a wok or skillet, over medium-high heat, heat the oil. Add the onion and celery and stir-fry for 3 minutes. Add the snow peas, water chestnuts, bamboo shoots, and stock. Cover and steam 1–2 minutes. Add the pepper and salt to taste. Snow peas should still be crisp and bright green when served.

Serves 6

Nutritive Information per Serving
Calories:                51
Protein (g):              3
Fat (g):                  2
Carbohydrates (g):        7

---

# SNACKS

## *Fruity Rice Cakes*

4 rice cakes
2 tbsp plus 2 tsp light cream cheese, softened
7 oz mandarin orange segments, drained
3/4 kiwi fruit, peeled and sliced
1/3 cup strawberries, sliced

Spread cream cheese over rice cakes and top with fruit.

Serves 4

Nutritive Information per Serving
Calories:                82
Protein (g):              3
Fat (g):                  2
Carbohydrates (g):       16

## *Fruit and Yogurt*

4 cups strawberries, hulled
1/2 lb pineapple chunks, drained and finely chopped
2 cups blueberry yogurt

Combine all ingredients in a bowl. Chill 10 minutes before serving.

Serves 6

Nutritive Information per Serving
Calories:                198

Protein (g):            7
Fat (g):                2
Carbohydrates (g):     41

### Grapple Pops

1/3 cup frozen grape juice concentrate, thawed
10 oz chunky applesauce
4 3-oz paper cups
4 wooden sticks

Combine juice and applesauce in a bowl and blend well. Fill each cup with about 1/3 cup juice mixture. Put cups in freezer. After about 1 hour of freezing, insert sticks. Freeze about 2 hours, or until firm. Remove cups to serve.

Serves 4

Nutritive Information per Serving
Calories:               88
Protein (g):            .6
Fat (g):                0
Carbohydrates (g):     21

# DRINKS

### Iced Zinger Tea

2 qt water
4 Red Zinger tea bags, or Lemon Zinger

Bring water to a boil in a heavy nonreactive saucepan. Add teabags and remove from heat. Cover pan and let stand 15–20 minutes to make a very strong tea. Let cool before serving. Pour over ice cubes. Sweeten with sugar or honey to taste.

Serves 4

Nutritive Information per Serving
Calories:                       0
Protein (g):                    0
Fat (g):                        0
Carbohydrates (g):              0

### Sage Tea

4 cups water
16 sage leaves, fresh or dried
1 tbsp plus 1 tsp sugar

Bring water to a boil. Add sage leaves and remove from heat. Let steep about 3 minutes, or longer if stronger tea is desired. Strain and serve sweetened with equal to taste.

Serves 4

Nutritive Information per Serving
Calories:                       16
Protein (g):                    0
Fat (g):                        0
Carbohydrates (g):              4

### Vegetable Orange Spritzer

2 cups low-sodium vegetable juice, chilled
1 cup plain or orange-flavored seltzer water, chilled
2 tbsp plus 2 tsp orange juice
4 orange slices

Combine first three ingredients. Serve over ice cubes. Garnish with orange slices.

Serves 4

Nutritive Information per Serving
Calories:                       45
Protein (g):                    1

Fat (g):                 0
Carbohydrates (g):       9

## *Ginger Tea*

1 tbsp plus 1 tsp black tea leaves
1/4 cup fresh ginger, thinly sliced
2 qt boiling water
1 tbsp plus 1 tsp sugar

Combine tea leaves and all but 4 ginger slices in a tea pot. Add boiling water and steep about 5 minutes. Strain tea into cups. Serve tea with a slice of ginger and sweeten to taste.

Serves 4

Nutritive Information per Serving
Calories:                20
Protein (g):             .1
Fat (g):                 0
Carbohydrates (g):       5

## *Creamy Tropical Shakes*

2 oranges, peeled and quartered
2 bananas, peeled
2 cups green or red seedless grapes
12 ice cubes, crushed
2 tsp honey
1/2 cup green or red seedless grapes, extra

Place first three ingredients in a blender or food processor and process until smooth. Add ice cubes and honey, and blend. Pour into glasses. Sprinkle with extra grapes as a garnish, if desired.

Serves 4

Nutritive Information per Serving
Calories:                193
Protein (g):             2

Fat (g):                        1
Carbohydrates (g):      49

## *Creamy Orange Fizz*

2/3 cup lowfat vanilla frozen yogurt
1 1/3 cups orange juice
1 tbsp plus 1 tsp confectioner's sugar
1 tbsp plus 1 tsp lemon juice
1/3 cup ice cubes
1 1/4 cups orange flavored sparkling water, chilled

Combine all ingredients, except sparkling water, in a blender.
Process until smooth. Combine orange juice mixture with
sparkling water in a pitcher. Stir until mixed thoroughly and serve.

Serves 4

Nutritive Information per Serving
Calories:                      80
Protein (g):                    2
Fat (g):                        0
Carbohydrates (g):      19

## *Strawberry Italian Ice*

4 cups strawberries, partially thawed if frozen
3/4 cup sugar
1/4 cup lemon juice
20 ice cubes

Place a large metal cake pan in freezer. Combine all ingredients,
except ice cubes, in a blender. Process until mixture is smooth and
sugar has dissolved. In batches if necessary, process strawberry
mixture with ice cubes until smooth. Pour into cake pan and freeze
30–35 minutes, or until partially frozen. Stir just before serving.

Serves 4

Nutritive Information per Serving
Calories:                195
Protein (g):               1
Fat (g):                   1
Carbohydrates (g):        49

---

# SPICES

## *Unbuttered Popcorn Topping*

1/2 tsp sea salt
1/4 cup plus 1 tbsp nutritional yeast

Grind salt with a mortar and pestle. Add yeast and grind. Sprinkle over freshly popped popcorn.

Serves 4

Nutritive Information per Serving
Calories:                 28
Protein (g):               4
Fat (g):                   0
Carbohydrates (g):         4

## *Quick Creole Spice*

1/2 tsp salt
1/4 tsp cayenne pepper
1/8 tsp finely ground black pepper
1/4 tsp dried basil
1/8 tsp dried thyme
1/4 tsp dried oregano
1/8 tsp garlic powder

Mix all ingredients and store in an air-tight container. Use as seasoning to taste.

Nutritive Information per Serving
Calories:                  1

Protein (g):              0
Fat (g):                  0
Carbohydrates (g):        .3


### Cranberry, Orange, and Apricot Salsa

3/4 cup fresh cranberries, coarsely chopped
2 tbsp honey
1 1/2 tsp fresh lime juice
1/4 small red onion, minced
1/2 jalapeño pepper, seeded and minced (wear rubber gloves)
1/2 large orange, peeled, segmented, seeded, and cut into 1/2 in.
    chunks
2 tbsp dried apricots, chopped
1 tbsp plus 1 tsp fresh cilantro, minced

Combine all ingredients in a mixing bowl. Chill overnight. Serve
over meat.

Serves 4

Nutritive Information per Serving
Calories:                 70
Protein (g):              1
Fat (g):                  0
Carbohydrates (g):        18


### Black Bean and Exotic Fruit Salsa

5 oz canned black beans, rinsed and drained
2 tbsp plus 2 tsp mango, peeled and cubed
2 tbsp plus 2 tsp papaya, peeled and diced
1/3 cup pineapple, cubed
2 tbsp plus 2 tsp red onion, diced
1/8 tsp habanero pepper sauce
1 tsp fresh cilantro, minced
1 tsp lime juice
1 tsp olive oil

1/4 tsp ground cumin
1/8 tsp salt
1/8 tsp black pepper
1 clove garlic, minced

Combine all ingredients in a large bowl and toss gently to coat. Let
stand 15 minutes before serving.

Serves 4

Nutritive Information per Serving
Calories:                  60
Protein (g):                3
Fat (g):                    2
Carbohydrates (g):         10

# *Appendix D*

# RESOURCES FOR GOOD HEALTH

## MINORITY HEALTH RESOURCES
### *Associations*

**www.personaldoc.com**

Provides personalized online health consultations with the author of this book, G. Edmond Smith, MD, M.Ed.

**National Black Woman's Health Project (NBWHP)**
1237 Ralph David Abernathy Blvd., SW
Atlanta, GA 30310
800-ASK-BWHP or 407-758-9590

**Black Women in Sports Foundation**
P.O. Box 2610
Philadelphia, PA 19130
215-763-6609

**National Institutes of Health Office of Research on Women**
Bldg. 1, Room 201
9000 Rockville Pike
Bethesda, MD 20892
301-402-2900

**Women's Health Network**
514 10th St., NW, Suite 400
Washington, DC 20004
202-347-1140
202-628-7814 (information line)
www.womenshealthnetwork.org

**Association for the Health Enrichment of Large People (AHELP)**
P.O. Drawer C
Radford, VA 24143
703-731-1778

**Weight Control Information Network**
1 Win Way
Bethesda, MD 20892-3665
301-984-7378
800-WIN-8098
win@info.niddk.nih.gov

**Eating Disorders Awareness Prevention (EDAP)**
603 Stewart Street, #803
Seattle, WA 98101
206-382-3587
www.edap.com

**The National Center for Overcoming Overeating**
315 W. 86th Street, #17-B
New York, NY 10024-3111
212-874-6596

**Food and Drug Administration**
5600 Fisher's Lane
Parklawn Bldg.
Rockville, MD 20857
888-INFO-FDA

**Melpomene Institute for Women's Health Research**
1010 University Avenue
St. Paul, MN 55104
612-642-1951

**National Organization for Women**
1000 16th St. NW
Washington, DC 10021
202-628-8669

**National Alliance of Breast Cancer Organizations**
9E 37th Street, 10th Floor
New York, NY 10016
800-719-9154
nabcoinfo@aol.com

**National Partnership for Women and Families**
1875 Connecticut Ave., NW, Suite 710
Washington, DC 20009
202-986-2600

**Young Women's Christian Association (YWCA)**
800-YWCA-US1 (call for your local chapter)

**Girls, Inc.**
30 East 33rd Street
New York, NY 10016
202-689-3700 (call for your local chapter)

**Hugs International**
P.O. Box 102A, RR3
Portage La Prairie, Manitoba Canada R1N3A3
800-565-4847

## Publications

### Healthy Weight Journal
Subscription Office:
Decker Periodicals, 4 Hughson Street South
P.O. Box 620 LCDI
Hamilton, ON, Canada L8N 3K7
800-568-7281
www.healthyweightnetwork.org

### Boston Women's Health Book Collective
Publishes: *Our Bodies, Ourselves*
240 A Elm Street
Somerville, MA 02144
617-628-3030
Info Center: 617-625-0271

### Health Wisdom for Women
Phillips Publishing, Inc.
7811 Montrose Road
P.O. Box 60110
Potomac, MD 20897-5924
800-804-0935

## Federal Offices

### The Office of Minority Health Resource Center
P.O. Box 37337
Washington, DC 20013-7337
800-444-6472

The Office of Minority Health Resource Center can provide information resources on minority health. Documents from the center are free and can be obtained by calling the number listed. Information can be obtained in English, Spanish, and Chinese.

### Centers for Disease Control and Prevention (CDC)
1600 Clifton Road, NE, Mail Stop D39

Atlanta, GA 30333
Fax: 404-639-2196

**Food and Drug Administration (FDA)**
Executive Director of Special Health Programs
Office of Consumer Affairs
Parklawn Building, Room 16-85
5600 Fishers Lane
Rockville, MD 20857
Fax: 301-443-9767

**National Institutes of Health**
Associate Director for Minority Programs
NIH Bldg. 31, Room 260
9000 Rockville Pike
Bethesda, MD 20892
Fax: 301-402-2517

**Substance Abuse and Mental Health Services Administration**
Associate Administrator for Minority Concerns
Rockwall II, Room 9D-18
5600 Fishers Lane
Rockville, MD 20857
Fax: 301-443-0526

---

# Ten U.S. Regions of the Public Health Service

**Public Health Service Region I**
Regional Program Consultant for Minority Health
John F. Kennedy Federal Building, Room 1826
Boston, MA 02203
States: CT, MA, ME, NH, RI, VT

**Public Health Service Region II**
Regional Program Consultant for Minority Health

26 Federal Plaza, Room 3337
New York, NY 10278
212-264-1324
States: NJ, NY, PR, U.S. Virgin Islands

**Public Health Service Region III**
Regional Minority Health Consultant
P.O. Box 13716, Mail Stop 14
3535 Market Street, Room 10200
Philadelphia, PA 19104
215-596-0487
States: DE, DC, MD, PA, VA, WV

**Public Health Service Region IV**
Regional Minority Health Consultant
101 Marietta Tower, Suite 1106
Atlanta, GA 30323
404-331-5917
States: AL, FL, GA, KY, MS, NC, SC, TN

**Public Health Service Region V**
Regional Minority Health Consultant
105 West Adams Street, 17th Floor
Chicago, IL 60603
312-353-0718
States: IL, IN, MI, MN, OH, WI

**Public Health Service Region VI**
Regional Minority Health Consultant
1200 Main Tower Building, Room 1800
Dallas, TX 75202
214-767-3871
States: AR, LA, NM, OK, TX

**Public Health Service Region VII**
Regional Minority Health Consultant
601 East Twelfth Street, Room 501

Kansas City, MO 64106
816-426-2178
States: IA, KS, MO, NE

**Public Health Service Region VIII**
Regional Minority Health Consultant
1961 Stout Street, Room 498
Denver, CO 80294
303-844-2019
States: CO, MT, ND, SD, UT, WY

**Public Health Service Region IX**
Regional Minority Health Consultant
50 United Nations Plaza, Room 327
San Francisco, CA 94102
415-556-3436
States: AZ, CA, HI, NV, American Samoa, Guam, Trust Territories
   of the Pacific Islands

**Public Health Service Region X**
Regional Program Consultant for Minority Health
2201 Sixth Avenue, Mail Stop RX-20
Seattle, WA 98121
206-615-2500
States: AK, ID, OR, WA

---

# State Minority Health Contacts

These states have official established offices for minority health. They are branches of the federal offices. If your state is not listed here, contact the federal office to determine your state's point of contact.

ALABAMA
Director
Minority Health Branch
Alabama Department of Public Health
11 South Union Street, Room 229

Montgomery, AL 36130-1701
205-613-5225

ARIZONA
Manager
Center for Minority Health, Room 005
Arizona Department of Health Services
1740 West Adams Street
Phoenix, AZ 85007
602-542-1025

ARKANSAS
Director
Office of Minority Health
Arkansas Department of Health
4815 West Markham Street-Slot 35
Little Rock, AR 72205
502-661-2193

CALIFORNIA
Chief
Office of Multicultural Health
California State Department of Health Services
601 North Seventh Street, MS-675
Sacramento, CA 95814
916-322-1519

DELAWARE
Minority Health Coordinator
Office of the Director
Delaware Health and Social Services
P.O. Box 637
Dover, DE 19903
302-739-4700

FLORIDA
Chairperson

Florida Commission on Minority Health
Florida A&M University
Ware-Rhaney Bldg., Room 103
Tallahassee, FL 32307
904-599-3817

GEORGIA
Director of Minority Health
Office of Policy and Planning
Division of Public Health
2 Peachtree Street, NW, Suite 203
Atlanta, GA 30302
404-657-2722

HAWAII
Administrator
Office of Hawaiian Health
State of Hawaii Department of Health
1250 Punch Bowl Street
Honolulu, HI 96813
808-586-4800

ILLINOIS
Director
Center for Minority Health
Illinois Department of Health
100 West Randolph, Suite 6-600
Chicago, IL 60601
312-814-5278

INDIANA
Director
Office of Special Populations
Indiana State Board of Health
1330 West Michigan Street, P.O. Box 1964
Indianapolis, IN 46206-1964
317-633-0100

LOUISIANA
Staff Director
Minority Health Affairs Council
State of Louisiana
Department of Health and Hospitals
P.O. Box 629
Baton Rouge, LA 70821-0629
504-342-9500

MASSACHUSETTS
Director
Office of Minority Health
Department of Public Health
150 Tremont Street, 10th Floor
Boston, MA 02111
617-727-7099

MICHIGAN
Chief
Office of Minority Health
Michigan Department of Public Health
3423 North Logan, P.O. Box 30195
Lansing, MI 48909
517-335-9287

MINNESOTA
Director
Office of Minority Health
Minnesota Department of Health
717 South East Delaware Street
P.O. Box 9441
Minneapolis, MN 55440
612-623-5794

MISSOURI
Chief
Office of Minority Health

State Department of Health
1738 East Elm Street, P.O. Box 570
Jefferson City, MO 65102
314-751-6064

NEBRASKA
Administrator
Office of Minority Health
Nebraska Department of Health
P.O. Box 95007
Lincoln, NE 86509-5007
402-471-2337

NEW JERSEY
Director
Office of Minority Health
State of New Jersey Department of Health-CN360
Trenton, NJ 08625-0369
609-292-6962

NEW YORK
Director
Office of Minority Health
New York State Department of Health
Empire State Plaza-Corning Tower, Room 1417
Albany, NY 12237-0601
518-474-2180

NORTH CAROLINA
Executive Director
Office of Minority Health
Environmental Health/Natural Resources
P.O. Box 27687
Raleigh, NC 27611-7687
919-733-7081

OHIO
Executive Director
Commission on Minority Health
77 South High Street, Suite 745
Vern Riffe Government Center
Columbus, OH 43266-0377
614-466-4000

OREGON
Manager
Minority Health Programs
Department of Human Resources
800 N.E. Oregon Street, #21
Portland, OR 97232
503-731-4582

RHODE ISLAND
Minority Health Coordinator
Office of Health Policy and Planning
Rhode Island Department of Health
Three Capitol Hill, Cannon, Room 408
Providence, RI 02908-5097
401-277-2901

SOUTH CAROLINA
Director
Office of Minority Health
Health and Environmental Control
2600 Bull Street
Columbia, SC 29201
803-734-4972

TENNESSEE
Director, Minority Health
Tennessee Department of Health
Tenn. Tower 312
8th Avenue North, 11th Floor

Nashville, TN 37219
615-741-7308

TEXAS
Director
Office of Minority Health
Texas Department of Health
1100 West Forty-Ninth Street
Austin, TX 78756-3179
512-458-7629

UTAH
Director
Ethnic Health Project
Department of Health
288 North 1460 West
Salt Lake City, UT 84116-0660
801-538-6129

VIRGINIA
Analyst for Minority Health
Office of the Commissioner
Virginia Department of Health
1500 East Main Street, Suite 213
Richmond, VA 23219
804-786-4891

U.S. VIRGIN ISLANDS
Acting Commissioner of Health
Office of the Commissioner
Virgin Islands Department of Health
Charles Harwood Hospital
3500 Richmond
Christiansed
St. Croix, VI 00820-4370
809-773-6551

# FEDERAL HEALTH INFORMATION CENTERS AND CLEARINGHOUSES

Listed here are clearinghouses for more information concerning the health and welfare of African Americans. These centers are equipped to answer questions concerning the specific topics outlined.

AGING
Alzheimer's Disease Education and Referral Center (ADEAR)
P.O. Box 8250
Silver Spring, MD 20907-8250
301-495-3311

National Elder Care Institute on Health Promotion
601 E Street, NW, 5th Floor
Washington, DC 20049
202-434-2200

National Center on Aging Information Center
P.O. Box 8057
Gaithersburg, MD 20898-8057
800-222-2225 or 800-222-4225 (TTY)

AIDS
CDC National AIDS Clearinghouse (NAC)
P.O. Box 6003
Rockville, MD 20850
800-458-5231 or 301-251-5160

ALCOHOL, DRUGS, SUBSTANCE ABUSE
CSAP National Clearinghouse for Alcohol and Drug Information
    (NCADI)
P.O. Box 2345
Rockville, MD 20847
800-729-6686 or 301-468-2600

CSAP National Resource Center for Prevention of Perinatal
    Substance Abuse
9302 Lee Highway
Fairfax, VA 22031
703-218-5700

ALLERGY AND INFECTIOUS DISEASES
National Institute of Allergy and Infectious Diseases (NIAID)
Building 31, Room 7A32
900 Rockville Pike
Bethesda, MD 20892
301-496-5717

ARTHRITIS
National Arthritis and Musculoskeletal and Skin Diseases
    Information Clearinghouse (NAMSIC)
9000 Rockville Pike, P.O. Box AMS
Bethesda, MD 20892
301-587-4352

BLINDNESS
National Library Service for the Blind and Physically Handicapped
    (NLSBPH)
Library of Congress
1291 Taylor Road, NW
Washington, DC 20542
202-707-0712

CANCER
Cancer Information Service (CIS)
National Cancer Institute (NCI)
Building 31, Room 10A16
9000 Rockville Pike
Bethesda, MD 20892
800-422-6237 or 301-469-5583

CHILD ABUSE
National Clearinghouse on Child Abuse and Neglect and Family
    Violence Information
3998 Fairridge Drive, Suite 350
Fairfax, VA 22033
800-394-3366 or 703-385-7565

CHILDREN AND YOUTH WITH HANDICAPS
National Information Center for Handicapped Children and Youth
    (NICHCY)
P.O. Box 1492
Washington, DC 20013
or 202-884-8200

CHRONIC DISEASE PREVENTION
Center for Disease Control and Prevention
Office of Public Enquiry
1600 Clifton Road, NE
Atlanta, GA 30333
404-639-3534

CONSUMER INFORMATION
Consumer Information Center
GSA, Room G142
Eighteenth & F Streets, NW
Washington, DC 20405
202-501-1794

Consumer Product Safety Commission Hotline (CPSC)
USCPSC
Washington, DC 20207
800-638-2772
800-638-8270 (AK, HI)
800-492-8104 (MD)

DEAFNESS
National Institute on Deafness and Other

Communication Disorders Clearinghouse (NIDCD)
1 Communications Drive
Bethesda, MD 20892
800-241-1044
800-241-1055 (TTY)

DENTAL RESEARCH
National Institute of Dental Research (NIDR)
Public Information Office
Building 31, Room 2C35
9000 Rockville Pike
Bethesda, MD 20892
301-496-4261

DIABETES
National Diabetes Information Clearinghouse (NDIC)
9000 Rockville Pike, P.O. Box NDIC
Bethesda, MD 20892
301-654-3327

DIGESTIVE DISEASES
National Digestive Diseases Information Clearinghouse (NDDIC)
9000 Rockville Pike, P.O. Box NDDIC
Bethesda, MD 20892
301-654-3810

DIRLINE
National Library of Medicine
8600 Rockville Pike
Bethesda, MD 20894
301-480-3537

DISABILITIES
Clearinghouse on Disability Information
OSERS/Department of Education
Switzer Building, Room 3132
400 Maryland Avenue, SW

Washington, DC 20202-2524
202-205-8412

EYE HEALTH
National Eye Institute (NEI)
Building 31, Room 6A32
9000 Rockville Pike
Bethesda, MD 20892
301-496-5248

FAMILY LIFE
Family Life Information Exchange (FLIE)
P.O. Box 37299
Washington, DC 20013-7299
301-585-6636

FOOD AND NUTRITION
Food and Nutrition Information Center (FNIC)
National Agricultural Library, Room 304
1301 Baltimore Boulevard
Beltsville, MD 20705-2351
301-504-5719

HEALTHCARE POLICY AND RESEARCH
AHCPR Publications Clearinghouse
P.O. Box 8547
Silver Springs, MD 20907-8547
or 301-495-3453

HEALTH PROMOTION AND DISEASE PREVENTION
ODPHP National Health Information Center (ONHIC)
P.O. Box 1133
Washington, DC 20013-1133
800-336-4797

HEART, LUNG AND BLOOD
NHLBI Education Programs Information Center

P.O. Box 30105
Bethesda, MD 20824-0105
301-251-1222

HUMAN SERVICES
Administration for Children and Families
370 L'Enfant Promenade, SW, 6th Floor West
Washington, DC 20447
202-401-9215

KIDNEY AND UROLOGIC DISEASES
National Kidney and Urologic Diseases Information Clearinghouse
(NKUDIC)
9000 Rockville Pike, P.O. Box NKUDIC
Bethesda, MD 20892
301-654-4415

MATERNAL AND CHILD HEALTH
National Center for Education in Maternal and Child Health
Clearinghouse
8201 Greensboro Drive, Suite 600
McLean, VA 22102
703-821-8955 (ext. 254/255)

MENTAL HEALTH
National Institute of Mental Health (NIMH)
Parklawn Building, Room 7C02
5600 Fishers Lane
Rockville, MD 20857
301-443-4513

MINORITY HEALTH
Office of Minority Health Resource Center (OMH-RC)
P.O. Box 37337
Washington, DC 20013-7337
301-587-1938

ORGAN TRANSPLANTATION
Health Resources and Services Administration (HRSA)
Division of Organ Transplantation
Parklawn Building, Room 7-18
5600 Fishers Lane
Rockville, MD 20857
301-443-7577

PHYSICAL FITNESS
President's Council on Physical Fitness and Sports
Market Square East Building, Suite 250
701 Pennsylvania Avenue, NW
Washington, DC 20004
202-272-3430

SECOND OPINION
National Second Surgical Opinion Hotline
200 Independence Avenue, SW
Washington, DC 20201
800-638-6833

SMOKING
Office on Smoking and Health (OSH)
Centers for Disease Control and Prevention MS K-50
4770 Buford Highway, NE
Atlanta, GA 30341
404-488-5707

---

# NATIONAL MINORITY ORGANIZATIONS

AFRICAN AMERICAN
National Black Women's Health Project
1237 Abernathy Boulevard, SW
Atlanta, GA 30310
404-758-9590

Association of Black Psychologists
821 Kennedy, NW
Washington, DC 20011
202-347-1895

National Medical Association
1012 Tenth Street, NW
Washington, DC 20001
202-393-6870

National Urban League, Inc. (NUL)
500 East Sixty-second Street
New York, NY 10021
212-310-9000

National Association of Black Social Workers, Inc. (NABSW)
15231 West McNichols
Detroit, MI 48235
313-862-6700

National Minority Health Association
P.O. Box 11876
Harrisburg, PA 17108-1876
717-761-1323

Black Congress on Health Law and Economics
1025 Connecticut Avenue, NW, Suite 610
Washington, DC 20036
202-659-4020

## SOURCES OF ADDITIONAL HEALTH MATERIAL FOR AFRICAN AMERICANS

American Association of Retired Persons
1909 K Street, NW
Washington, DC 20049
202-434-2277

American Cancer Society
3340 Peachtree Road NE
Atlanta, GA 30026
800-227-2345

American Diabetes Association
National Service Center
1660 Duke Street
Alexandria, VA 22314
703-549-1500

American Heart Association National Center
7320 Greenville Avenue
Dallas, TX 75231
214-373-6300

American Lung Association
1740 Broadway
New York, NY 10019-4374
800-LUNG-USA

CDC National AIDS Clearinghouse
P.O. Box 6003
Rockville, MD 20849-6003
800-458-5231

Institute on Black Chemical Dependency
2616 Nicollet Avenue South
Minneapolis, MN 55408
612-871-7878

March of Dimes Birth Defects Foundation
1275 Mamaroneck Avenue
White Plains, NY 10605
914-428-7100

Minority AIDS Project
5149 West Jefferson Boulevard
Los Angeles, CA 90016
213-936-4949

National Association for Equal Opportunity in Higher Education
Black Higher Education Center
Lovejoy Building
400 Twelfth Street, NE
Washington, DC 20002
202-543-9111

National Black Child Development Institute, Inc.
1023 Fifteenth Street, NW
Washington, DC 20005
202-387-1281

# References

*American Psychiatric Association: Diagnostic and Statistical Manual of Mental Disorders: DSM-IV*, 4th ed. Washington D.C., American Psychiatric Association, 1994.

Arnold, J. "Move It or Lose It, Flexibility: It's the Key to Vitality," *My Generation*, May–June 2001, pp. 20–24.

Barefoot, J. C., Schroll, M. "Symtoms of Depression, Acute Myocardial Infarction, and Total Mortality in a Community Sample," *Circulation*, 1996: 93 (11):1976–1980.

Benjamin, S., et al. "Mind-Body Medicine: Expanding the Health Model," *Patient Care*, Sept 15 1997, pp. 127–142.

Blazer, D. G., Kessler, R. C., McGonayle, K. A., et al. "The Prevalence and Distribution of Major Depression in a National Community Sample: The National Comorbidity Survey," *Am J Psychiatry*, 1994; 151 (7):979–986.

Bonow, R.O., Bohannon, N., Hazzard, W. "Risk Stratification in Coronary Artery Disease and Special Populations," *AM J Med*, 1996; 101 (suppl 4A):175–245.

Brill, P. A., Giles, W. H., Keenan, N. L., et al. "Effect of Body Mass Index Activity Limitation and Mortality Among Older Women: The National Health Interview Survey," 1986–1990. *J Women's Health*, 1997; 6 (4):435–440.

Byrne, A., Byrne, D.G. "The Effect of Exercise on Depression,

Anxiety and Mood States: A Review." *J Psychosom Res,* 1993; 37 (6):565–574.

Calloway, D. H., Havel, R. J., Bier, D. M., et al. *Nutrition and Your Health: Dietary Guidelines for Americans,* 4th ed. U.S. Government Printing Office: 1996-402-519, U.S. Dept of Health and Human Services, U.S. Dept. of Agriculture, 1995, Washington, D.C.

"Clinical Guidelines on the Identification, Evaluation, and Treatment of Overweight and Obesity in Adults," *The Evidence Report.* National Institutes of Health. Bethesda, MO: National Heart, Lung, and Blood Institute of Diabetes and Digestive and Kidney Diseases, 1998. NIH Publication 98-4083.

Committee on Diet and Health; Food and Nutrition Board, "Diet and Health: Implications for Reducing Chronic Disease Risk" (Washington, D.C.: National Academy Press, 1989), pp. 563–592.

Criek, P. J., Sherer, J. T., Stier, Carson D. "Management of Obesity: Medical Treatment Options," *American Family Physician,* 1997, 55:551–558.

Crouch, M.A., ed. "Effective Use of Statins to Prevent Coronary Heart Disease," *American Family Physician,* January 15, 2000, Vol. 63, No. 2.

Dell, D. L., Stewart, D. E. "Menopause and Mood: Is Depression Linked with Hormone Changes?" *Post Gradate Medicine,* Vol. 108, No. 3, Sept 2000, pp. 34–43.

Dougherty, R. M., Fong, A. K., Iacono, J. M. "Nutrient Content of the Diet When the Fat Is Reduced." *American Journal of Clinical Nutrition,* 1988, 48: 970–979.

Flink, E. B. "Magnesium Deficiency: Etiology and Clinical Spectrum," *Acta Med Scand,* 1981: 674 (suppl):125–137.

Goleman, D. *Emotional Intelligence.* Bantam Book, 1995.

Grandjean, A. C. "Dietary Strategies for Modifying Weight or Body Composition, Strength and Conditioning," *Medicine & Science in Sports and Exercise,* 1995, 17(3):7–10.

"Health and Behavior: Personality Has Effect on AIDS; High Stress Makes You Prone to Colds; Mate Influences Your Blood Pressure," *USA Today,* March 13, 2001, 70.

Hyman, Bradley. "Protein Clears Alzheimer's Plaque on Brains of Mice," *The Journal Nature Medicine*, March 2001.

Jing, A., Folsom, A., Melnick, S. A., et al. "Association of Serum and Dietary Magnesium with Cardiovascular Disease, Hypertension, Diabetes, Insulin and Carotid Wall Thickness: The ARIC Study," *J Clin Epidemiol*, 1995, 48:927–940.

Kushner R., Hopson S. "Obesity Therapy: What Works-What Doesn't," *Consultant Journal*, March 1998, 511–518.

Lobo R. A., ed. *Treatment of the Postmenopausal Woman: Basic and Clinical Aspects.* New York, NY: Raven Press LTD, 1994.

Lukaski, A. C. "Magnesium, Zinc, and Chromium Nutrition and Physical Activity," *American Journal of Clinical Nutrition*, 2000, 72 (suppl):5855–5935.

Mahler, D. A. *American College of Sports Medicine: Guidelines for Exercise Testing and Prescription*, 5th ed. Baltimore, Williams and Wilkins, 1995, pp. 1–37.

Matthews, K. A., Meilahn, E., Kuller, L. H., et al. "Menopause and Risk Factors for Coronary Heart Disease," *New England Journal of Medicine*, 1989, 321 (10):641–646.

Miller, W. C. "How Effective Are Traditional Dietary and Exercise Intervention for Weight Loss?" *Medicine & Science in Sports and Exercise*, 1999, 31 (8):1, 129–131,134.

Moser, M. "Management of Hypertension: Part 11," *American Family Physician*, June 1996: 53:2553–2560.

National Institutes of Health Consensus Development Conference. *Health Implications of Obesity*, February 1985.

National Institutes of Health. *Clinical Guidelines on the Identification, Evaluation, and Treatment of Overweight and Obesity in Adults.* Betheseda, MD: U.S. Dept of Health and Human Services, 1998. NIH Publication No. 98-4083.

*New Analyses Regarding the Safety of Calcium Channel Blockers*; A Statement for Health Professionals from the National Heart, Lung and Blood Institute. Bethesda, MD: National Institutes of Health, 1995.

*Nutrition in Exercise and Sport*, 3rd ed. Boca Raton, Fl. CRC Press, 1998.

Poehlman, E. T., Toth, M. J., Gardner, A. W. "Changes in Energy

Balance and Body Composition at Menopause: A Controlled Longitudinal Study," *Ann Intern Med*, 1995, 123(9):673–675.

Regal, K. M., Carroll, M. D., Kuczmarski, R. J., et al. "Overweight and Obesity in the United States—Prevalence and Trends, 1960–1994," *Int. J. Obes Relat Metab Disord*, 1998, 22: 39–47.

Revven, Baron. "The Development of a Concept of Psychological Well-Being," Ph.D. dissertation, Rhodes University, South Africa, 1988.

Shahady, E. "Exercise as Medication: How to Motivate Your Patients." *Consultant*, November 2000, pp. 2174–2177.

Simkin-Silverman, L. R., Wing, R. R. "Management of Obesity in Primary Care," *Obes Res*, 1997, 5(6):603–612.

Simkin-Silverman, L. R., Wing, R. R., Boraz, M. A., et al. "A Randomized Clinical Trial of Weight Gain Prevention in 535 Healthy Women During Menopause," *Circulation*, 1999, 100 (18):1–238.

Snelling, A., Begany, T. "Nutrition Counseling," *Patient Care*, April 30, 1997, 47–53.

Statistics from Harris Poll; Henry J. Kaiser Family Foundation/ Harvard School of Public Health.

Stern, M. "Epidemiology of Obesity and Its Link to Heart Disease." *Metabolism*, 1995, 44(9) (suppl 3):1–3.

Turczn, K. M., Klein, R. J., Schnobler, S. E., et al. *Healthy People 2000; Natural Health Promotion and Disease Prevention Objectives: Healthy People 2000 Review* 1995-96, DHHS Publication No. (PHS) 95-1256-1. U.S. Dept of Health and Human Service, Centers for Disease Control and Prevention, National Center for Health Statistics, 1996, Hyattsville, MD.

Under, A. C., Nieman, D. C., Shannonhouse, E. M., et al. "Influence of Diet and/or Exercise on Body Composition and Cardiorespiratory Fitness in Obese Women," *International Journal of Sport Nutrition*, 1998, 8: 213–222.

U.S. Department of Health and Human Services. *Physical Activity and Health: A Report of the Surgeon General.* Atlanta, DHHS, Centers for Disease Control and Prevention, National Center for Chronic Disease Prevention and Health Promotion, 1996.

Van Staa, T. P., ed. "Use of Statins and Risk of Fractures," *JAMA*, 2001, 285:1850–1855.

Weinsier, R. L., et al. "Energy Expenditure and Free-Living Physical Activity in Black and White Women," *AMJ Clin Nutrition*, 2000, 71:1138–1146.

Weissman, M. M., Bland, R., Joyce, P. R., et al. "Sex Differences in Rates of Depression: Cross-Natural Perspectives," *J Affect Disord*, 1993, 29 (2-3):77–84.

Whang, R., Hampton, E. M., Whang, D. D. "Magnesium Homeostasis and Clinical Disorders of Magnesium Deficiency," *Ann Pharmacother*, 1994, 28:220–226.

Wing, R. R., Matthews, K. A., Kuller, L. H., et al. "Weight Gain at the Time of Menopause," *Arch Intern Med*, 1991, 151 (1):97–102.

# Subject Index

abdominal training (exercises), 133–137
acceptance of others, as positive change, 22
Africa
  average African diet, 12
  traditional foods of, 12
African American women
  and diabetes, 4
  and heart disease, fatalities caused by, 4, 5
  knowing themselves, 21–23
  and obesity, 5, 17, 47–48
  and "sisterhood" as source of support, 64, 167
  troubling facts about health, 5
  why reluctant to lose weight, 8
African Americans
  and cultural history of foods, 11–12
  and slavery, diet of, 13–14
  effect of industrial revolution on diet, 16
anger, learning to handle, 109–111
assertiveness, using in positive manner, 120–122
  rules of, 121–122

balance, finding in life, 9
Benson, Dr. Herbert, and Relaxation Response, 185
bibliography, 353–357
BMI. *See* Body Mass Index
Body Mass Index (BMI)
  calculating your own, 247–249
  using to determine if overweight, 7, 47
breathing exercise, as part of mental warm-up, 39

calories
  counting, 102
  exchange lists (1,200–2,500), 228–232
  foods low in (less then 20 calories), 245–246
  healthy attitude towards, 194
  number burned by various exercises, 132
  recommended intake of, 87
carbohydrates
  complex, 51
  exchange list, 233–235
  facts about, 51–52, 84
  how our bodies use, 52

myth surrounding, 57–58
change, stages of, 126–128
cholesterol, 55
  high cholesterol and heart disease, 141–142
  lowering, 139–140
coping mechanisms, list of positive, 124

depression, 143–144
  Prozac and, 143
  symptoms of, 144
desserts (exchange list), 243
diabetes, and African American women, 4
diary, keeping a, 194
  daily food diary (form), 259
diet sodas, not overdoing, 122
dieting. *See also* weight loss
  as fad, 63–64
  finding support for, 64
  misconceptions about, 3
  negative connotation about the word 'diet', 50
  yo-yo dieting, 64
doctor-patient relationship, developing a good, 32, 36
doctors. *See also* family medicine
  finding one you're comfortable with, 31, 34–36
  importance of being culturally sensitive, 33
  organization of African American doctors, 34, 349
dumbbells (exercise equipment)
  exercising with, 101–102, 108, 251–256

eating disorders, questionnaire to identify a problem, 173–175
eating habits, changing a lifetime of, 10

eating well
  healthy ways of eating, 194–197
  list of strategies for, 130–132
emotional fitness
  benefits of, 37, 41–43, 44, 46
  learning to delay gratification, 44–45
  mental warm-up, 39–41
  and obesity, 46–48
  steps to getting started, 38
  and weight loss, 42–43
emotional fitness inventory, 88–89, 175–182
  emotional inventory questionnaire, 176–177
  physical inventory questionnaire, 177–179
  social inventory questionnaire, 179–181
  stress inventory questionnaire, 181–182
emotional support, finding with other women, 28
  concept of "sisterhood", 28, 31–32, 64, 167
ephedra (herb), using to help with weight loss, 90
exchange lists, 228–247
  breads, 234
  carbohydrates, 233–235
  cereals/grains/pastas, 233
  combination foods, 244–245
  crackers/snacks, 234–235
  desserts, 243
  dried beans/peas/lentils, 233
  fast foods, 244
  fat, 241–243
  free foods (less then 20 calories), 245–246
  fruits, 235–237
  meat, 239–241
  milk, 238–239

starch foods, prepared with fat, 235
starchy vegetables, 234
vegetables, 237–238
exercise. *See also* strength training
abdominal muscle exercises, 133–137
aerobic activity log, 260
calories burned by various, 132
dumbbells, 101–102, 108, 251–256
finding motivation to, 99–100
flexibility stretching exercises, 144–149
lack of time as poor excuse for not exercising, 59–60
low-impact, 145
muscle cramps, relieving, 152–153
push-ups, 253, 256
standing leg presses, 255
walking, 88, 100, 108, 132–133

family medicine. *See also* doctors
finding family doctor you're comfortable with, 30, 34–35
historical model of, 29
need for culturally sensitive doctors, 33
role family doctor plays, 29, 30
fast food (exchange list), 244
fat (exchange list), 241–243
saturated fats, 242–243
unsaturated fats, 242
fats
burning off, 56, 87–88
cholesterol and, 55
"essential" fatty acids, 53
facts about, 53–54, 85–86
monounsaturated, 54
myth about, 59
saturated, 53, 54, 242–243

triglycerides and, 55
unsaturated, 53, 242
fiber, importance of, 113
food cravings
caused by stress, 105–106
trigger foods, 130, 140–141
food exchange lists. *See* exchange lists
fruits (exchange list), 235–237
dried fruit, 236
fresh, frozen, and unsweetened, 235–236
fruit juice, 236–237

goals
becoming goal-oriented, 8, 37–38
becoming self-aware, 44
for women on wellness journey, 76
grocery list, healthy (checklist), 262–263
gym, getting motivated about going, 40–41

health insurance, four types of, 35
health literacy, what is, 50–51
healthy habits, tips for achieving, 191–193
heart disease
and African American women, 4
and high cholesterol, 141–142
and obesity, 143
high blood pressure, 142
hypertension. *See* high blood pressure

impulse control, tips for, 43–44

journal keeping, as way of knowing yourself, 23–25, 99

knee problems, caused by overexercising, 144–145
knowing yourself, 21–23
keeping a journal as tool for,
23–25

liposuction (surgical procedure),
129–130

magnesium deficiency, 152–153
foods high in magnesium, 153
medical conditions related to,
152–153
meal plan (sample weekly)
daily food diary, 259
exchange list (by calories in
1200–2,500 range), 228–232
Week 1, 199–205
Week 2, 205–211
Week 3, 212–218
Week 4, 218–224
weekly calendar, 258
meals
eating lots of small, 87, 112
healthy eating habits, 196–197
not skipping, 194
meat, eating, and myth about,
58–59
meat (exchange list)
high-fat meat and substitutes,
241
lean meat and substitutes,
239–240
medium-fat meat and substitutes, 240–241
meditation
benefits of, 183–184
having a regular time for,
188–189
how to, 186–187
meditation exercise, 96–99
for relaxation, 89

spiritual aspects of, 186
for stress reduction, 184–185
using a mantra, 188
what is, 183
menopause, 150–151
sexuality and, 150–151
mental imagery, as part of mental
warm-up, 39–40
metabolism, speeding up
caution regarding using a quick-
fix, 89–90
milk (exchange list), 238–239
skim/lowfat, 238–239
whole, 239
mind-body component of weight
loss, 168–169
misconceptions about wellness,
197–198
motivation, finding to lose weight,
86
muscle cramps, from exercising,
152–153

negative thoughts, examples of
common, 24
nutrition, being literate about,
50–51

obesity
African American women and,
5, 17, 47–48
calculating with Body Mass
Index, 47
emotional fitness and, 46–48
epidemic of, 5, 47–48
and heart disease, 143
medical definition, 46
premature deaths attributed to,
48
osteoporosis, 151
lowering risk for, 151
overtraining, signs of, 117

personal narratives (of women in
   weight loss program), 76
  Diane (35 year-old church secretary), 67–70
  in a nutshell, 77
  testimony to the benefits of the
   program, 160–162
  Rose (30 year-old pharmacy
   technician), 70–74
  in a nutshell, 77
  testimony to the benefits of the
   program, 163–165
  Tameka (52 year-old lawyer),
   74–76
  in a nutshell, 77
  testimony to the benefits of the
   program, 165–167
  Tawanda (20 year-old college
   student), 65–67
  in a nutshell, 76–77
  testimony to the benefits of program, 155–160
personality, defined, 22
personality "pie" (major personality traits), 8, 25–27
  intellectual, 26
  mental/emotional, 26
  physical/sexual, 26
  social, 27
  spiritual, 27
positive affirmations, list of, 24
positive attitude about wellness,
   maintaining, 102
positive ways to achieve wellness,
   191–193
  healthy ways of acting, 194–197
potassium supplements, 153
protein
  excellent sources of, 53, 103–104
  facts about, 52–53, 83
Prozac (medication), 143
publications on wellness, 332

relaxation
  forms of active, 124
  Relaxation Response and, 185
  using meditation for, 185
resources
  Federal health information centers & clearinghouses,
   342–348
  Federal offices, 332–333
  minority health, 329–331,
   349–351
  National Medical Association,
   34, 349
  national minority organizations,
   348–349
  Public Health Services (U.S.
   regional offices), 333–335
  publications, 332
  State Minority health contacts,
   335–341
  Website of author, 329
responsibility, taking for wellness,
   49


salt intake, limiting, 87
seasonings, list of, 246–247
self-awareness, as goal, 44
self-expression, important steps to,
   110
shape, how your body loses (illus-
   tration), 175
"sisterhood", finding support
   among, 64, 167
slavery in America, and impact on
   diet, 13–15
  health problems as result of
   high-fat diet, 15–16
sleep
  importance of getting sufficient,
   116–117
  sleep deprivation and weight
   gain, 117

snacks, healthy, 88
  caution about, 122–123
sodium. *See* salt
"soul food", origins of, 11–12
  and Civil Rights movement, 16
starch foods. *See* carbohydrates
stomach
  exercises that burn fat off,
    122–137
  liposuction, 129–130
  making flatter, 129
strength training, 100–102. *See
  also* exercise
  benefits of, 100–101
  dumbbells, working out with,
    101–102, 108, 251–256
  strength training log (form), 261
stress
  handling, 42
  meditation to relieve, 184–185
  stress inventory questionnaire,
    181–182
  toll it takes on emotional health,
    38
stretching exercises for flexibility,
  146–149
  back and chest (crossover
    stretch), 146
  chest and shoulders (arm cir-
    cles), 147
  hips (quad stretch and hip
    opener), 149
  legs and hip joints (hamstring
    stretch), 148
  neck and spine (back arch),
    147
Sunday dinners, origins of, 15–
  16
supplements. *See* vitamins and
  supplements
symptoms, telling doctor both
  physical and emotional, 32

thinking, unhealthy ways of,
  197–198
time management, having for daily
  activities, 46
trigger foods, 130. *See also* food
  cravings
  substitutes for, 130, 140–141

unhealthy eating, controlling
  impulses, 43–44

vegetables (exchange list), 237–238
vitamins and supplements
  importance of, 87
  myth that taking vitamins will
    make you fat, 58, 87
  potassium supplements, 153
  supplements for magnesium
    deficiency, 153

Walker, Alice (author)
  coined term "womanist", 4
  quote, 3
walking (exercise), 88, 100
  calories expended by, 132
  tips for better workout, 132–133
  with partner, 108
water
  importance of drinking lots of,
    85, 95–96, 102–103, 195
  myth that drinking will cause
    you to gain weight, 57
weight loss. *See also* dieting
  eating at defined times, 112
  importance of emotional fitness
    and motivation, 42–43
  nutritional myths about, 56–60
  pills not the answer, why, 90
  programs
  amount spent annually on, 6
  showing before and after pic-
    tures, 125

why most don't work, 6
stages of change, 126–128
supplements to help with, 90
why most attempts fail, 112–113
Weight Loss Program (Week 1)
emotional inventory, 88–89
finding motivation to be on program, 86
first meeting, 79
fundamentals for Week 1, 90–91
importance of good nutrition,
83–85
importance of teamwork, 86
initial weight of women, 80
picking a partner, 80–81
reasons for joining the wellness
program, 81–83
sample meal plan, 199–205
Weight Loss Program (Week 2)
awareness about foods, 94
calorie counting, 102
drinking lots of water, importance of, 95–96, 102–103
exercising with a partner, 94–95
finding motivation to exercise,
99–100
fundamentals for Week 2, 104
high-protein foods, eating,
103–104
journal keeping, 99
meditation exercise, 96–99
positive attitude, maintaining a,
102
sample meal plan, 205–211
strength training, 100–102
walking, 100
weight loss recorded for the
week, 93
Weight Loss Program (Week 3)
anger, learning to handle,
109–111
eating at defined times, 112

emotional health, importance
of, 108–109
energy levels, increase in,
107–108
food cravings, 105
fundamentals for Week 3, 113
sample meal plan, 212–218
tip to help drink more water,
106–107
walking with partner, 108
weight loss recorded for the
week, 105
Weight Loss Program (Week 4)
assertive, learning to be,
120–122
blood cholesterol levels, 115–
116
changes should be made slowly,
116
fundamentals for Week 4,
123–124
positive coping mechanisms, 124
sample meal plan, 218–224
setting boundaries with family,
118–119
signs of overtraining, 117
sleeping properly, 116–117
weight loss recorded for the
week, 115
Weight Loss Program (Week 5)
exercises listed by calories
expended, 132
fundamentals for Week 5,
137–138
showing before and after pictures, 125
stages of change, 126–128
strategies for eating well,
130–132
tightening the belly, 129–130,
133–137
tips for walking, 132–133

weight loss recorded for the week, 125

Weight Loss Program (Week 6)
cholesterol levels, lowering, 139–140
depression, 143–144
fundamentals for Week 6, 153–154
heart disease and obesity, 143
high blood pressure, 142
high cholesterol, 141–142
knee problems, from overexercising, 144–145
menopause, 150–151
muscle cramps, relieving, 152–153
osteoporosis, lowering the risk for, 151–152
stretching exercises, 146–149
total weight loss for women, 139

Weight Loss Program (Week 7)
fundamentals for Week 7, 162
testimony of women on benefits of program, 155–160, 160–162

total weight loss for women, 155

Weight Loss Program (Week 8)
final thoughts, 167–169
testimony of women on benefits of program, 163–165, 165–167
total weight loss for women, 163

weight training. See strength training

wellness
emotional fitness and, 37–41
finding support with "sisterhood", 64, 167
goals for women on journey to, 76
Hippocrates on, 4
mind-body component, 168–169
misconceptions about, 197–198
positive ways to achieve, 191–193, 194–197
setting clearly defined boundaries, 118–119
taking responsibility for, 49

# Recipe Index

Asparagus with Italian Dressing, 304

Baked Cod, 281
Baked Potatoes, 304–305
Barbecued Chicken Breasts,
   281–282
Bean Salad, South-of-the-Border,
   277–278
Bell Peppers and Mushrooms,
   305–306
Black Bean & Exotic Fruit Salsa,
   326–327
Broccoli Tomatoes Sauté, 312
Broccoli with Italian Dressing, 304
Broccoli with Lemon, 308
Brown-Rice and Mushroom Soup
   (slow cooker), 275
Buttered Green Beans, 311

Cajun Chicken Breasts (grill
   machine), 283
Cauliflower Soup (slow cooker),
   274–275
Caesar Salad, 279
Chicken Alphabet Soup, 279–280
Chicken Casserole, 294–295
Chicken Divan, 295–295
Chicken Provencal, 296

Chicken Salad, 272
Chicken Vegetable Stir Fry, 297–298
Chicken with Lemon Thyme
   Sauce, 298–299
Chilled Potatoes in Creamy Herb
   Sauce, 315–316
Cod with Orange Sauce, 282–283
Cold Tomato Soup, 276
Crab Louis, 299
Cranberry, Orange & Apricot
   Salsa, 326
Creamy Carrots and Peas, 310
Creamy Cucumber Salad, 271
Creamy Orange Fizz, 324
Creole Spice (Quick), 325–326
Crystal Shrimp with Sweet & Sour
   Sauce, 300–301
Curried Carrots, 314
Curried Waldorf Salad, 270–271

French Toast, New Zealand,
   268–269
Fruit and Yogurt, 320–321

Ginger Tea, 323
Grapple Pops, 321
Green Beans in Mustard, 309
Grilled Chicken Breasts, 301

Grilled Pineapple Slices, 266
Grilled Shrimp with Pasta &
    Pineapple Salsa, 291–292

Halibut in Foil, 292–293

Ice Zinger Tea, 321–322

Lemon Carrots, 313, 318
Lemon Chicken, 301–302
Lemon Dijon Chicken, 287–288
Lemon Green Beans, 315

Maple Beans, 309–310
Mashed Potatoes, 312–313
Miso Soup (microwave), 274
Mixed Salad, 271–272
Mustard Grilled Turkey Breasts,
    288–289

Oatmeal, Fruity (microwave), 268

Pancakes (egg-white), 269
Pasta and Salmon Salad, 284
Penne with Chicken, Peas, and
    Peppers, 289
Poached Flounder, 285
Pork Filet with Mustard-
    Peppercorn Sauce, 282
Pork Picante, Peachy, 290
Potato Salad, Herbed, 316
Potato Salad, Mom's, 272–273
Pumpkin Muffins (fat-free),
    266–267
Red Chicken with Almonds, 302–303
Red Snapper (pan-fried), 290
Rice Cakes, Fruity, 320
Rice with Peas, 311
Roast Pork, 284
Roasted Vegetable Soup, 276–277

Sage Tea, 322
Shrimp Rémoulade, 303–304

Snow Peas with Water Chestnuts
    & Bamboo Shoots, 319–320
Spaghetti Squash (baked), 317–318
Steamed Cabbage, 307
Steamed Carrots, 308–309
Strawberry Italian Ice, 324–325
Stuffed Bell Peppers, 307–308
Stuffed Chicken Breasts, 285–286

Tarragon Asparagus, 313–314
Texas Chili, 278
Thousand Island Dressing, 271–272
Tropical Fruit Cup, 266
Tropical Shake, Creamy, 267–268,
    323–324
Turkey Breast Sandwich, 269–270
Turkey Fillets with Apple Rum,
    280–281
Turkey Fillets with Lemon and
    Sage, 286–287
Turkey Provencal, 293–294
Turkey Sandwich with Cranberry-
    Orange-Relish, 273
Turkey Tortilla Soup (slow
    cooker), 291

Unbuttered Popcorn Topping, 325

Veal Cutlets, 286
Vegetable Basket (grilled), 318–319
Vegetable Medley, Quick, 317
Vegetable Orange Spritzer, 322–323
Vegetable Stew (lowfat), 306

BREAKFAST (recipes), 265–269

DINNER (recipes), 280–304

DRINKS (recipes)
Creamy Orange Fizz, 324
Creamy Tropical Shakes, 267–268,
    323–324
Ginger Tea, 323

Ice Zinger Tea, 321–322
Sage Tea, 322
Strawberry Italian Ice, 324–325
Vegetable Orange Spritzer, 322–323

LUNCH (recipes), 269–280

SALADS (recipes)
Black Bean & Exotic Fruit Salsa,
    326–327
Caesar Salad, 279
Chicken Salad, 272
Creamy Cucumber Salad, 271
Curried Waldorf Salad, 270–271
Herbed Potato Salad, 316
Mom's Potato Salad, 272–273
Pasta and Salmon Salad, 284
South-of-the-Border Bean Salad,
    277–278
Thousand Island Dressing, 271–272

SANDWICH (recipes)
Turkey Breast, 269–270
Turkey Sandwich with Cranberry-
    Orange Relish, 273

SNACKS (recipes)
Fruit and Yogurt, 320–321
Fruity Rice Cakes, 320
Grapple Pops, 321

SOUPS (recipes)
Chicken Alphabet Soup, 279–280
Cold Tomato Soup, 276
Lowfat Vegetable Stew, 306
Microwave Miso Soup, 274
Roasted Vegetable Soup, 276–277
Slow Cooker Brown-Rice &
    Mushroom Soup, 275
Slow Cooker Cauliflower Soup,
    274–275
Slow Cooker Turkey Tortilla Soup,
    291

Zesty Texas Chili, 278

SPICES (recipes)
Black Bean & Exotic Fruit Salsa,
    326–327
Cranberry, Orange & Apricot
    Salsa, 326
Quick Creole Spice, 325–326
Unbuttered Popcorn Topping, 325

VEGETABLE SIDE DISHES
    (recipes)
Asparagus with Italian Dressing,
    305
Baked Potatoes, 304–305
Baked Spaghetti Squash, 317–318
Broccoli Tomatoes Sauté, 312
Broccoli with Italian Dressing, 304
Broccoli with Lemon, 308
Buttered Green Beans, 311
Chilled Potatoes in Creamy Herb
    Sauce, 315–316
Cooked Peppers & Mushrooms,
    305–306
Creamy Carrots and Peas, 310
Curried Carrots, 314
Golden Mashed Potatoes, 312–313
Green Beans in Mustard, 309
Grilled Vegetable Basket, 318–319
Herbed Potato Salad, 316
Lemon Green Beans, 315
Light Lemon Carrots, 313
Lowfat Vegetable Stew, 306
Maple Beans, 309–310
Microwave Lemon Carrots, 313,
    318
Quick Vegetable Medley, 317
Rice with Peas, 311
Snow Peas with Water Chestnuts
    & Bamboo Shoots, 319–320
Steamed Carrots, 308–309
Stuffed Bell Peppers, 307–308
Tarragon Asparagus, 313–314